Proceedings of the
Ninth International Congress on
Hyperbaric Medicine

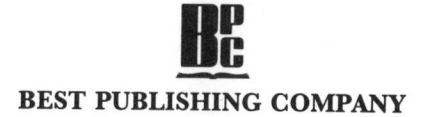

BEST PUBLISHING COMPANY

Proceedings of the Ninth International Congress on
Hyperbaric Medicine

President: Ian P. Unsworth, M.D.
        Sydney, Australia

Secretariat: Frederick S. Cramer, M.D.
        San Francisco, U.S.A.

March 1-4, 1987
Sydney, Australia

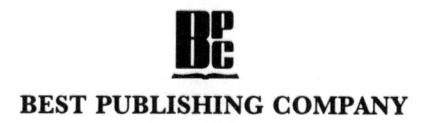

BEST PUBLISHING COMPANY

All rights reserved

No part of this book may be reproduced, stored in a retrieval system, or transmitted in any form or by any means, electronic, mechanical, photocopying, microfilm, recording, or otherwise, without permission from the publisher

Copyright © 1998, by Best Publishing Company

Printed and bound in the United States of America

Proceedings of the Ninth International Congress on Hyperbaric Medicine

International Standard Book Number
ISBN 0-941332-34-9

Library of Congress Catalog Card Number
93-070913

Published By
Best Publishing Company
Post Office Box 30100
Flagstaff, AZ 86003-0100

CONTENTS

Foreword — ix

Proceedings of the IX International Congress on Hyperbaric Medicine — xi

Air and fat emboli in the lung and the brain; *B. A. Hills* — 1

Changes of rat spinal evoked potentials in acute decompression sickness; *Xu Tie Supervisor: Prof. Ni Guo-Tan* — 7

Control of HPNS with trimix 5 (5% N_2/He/O_2) to 600 m; *Peter B. Bennett, Richard D. Vann, Henry Schafstall, J. Holthaus and W. Schnegelsberg* — 11

Change in lung diffusion capacity (LDC) during acute decompression sickness (DCS) in awake rabbits; *Jiang Jian-Yong, Supervisor: Prof. Ni Guo-Tan* — 23

Treatment of decompression sickness hawaiian style; *Frank P. Farm, Jr., Edwin Hayashi, Edward L. Beckman, M.D.* — 27

Changes of volume, K+, Na+, Cl-, and 17-OHCS of human urine during the simulated short-term air diving in dry chamber; *G. T. Ni and H. J. Chen* — 33

An investigation for evaluation of different recompression treatment tables of air decompression sickness by means of agarose gel bubble technique; *Hang, Rong-Chung Lian and Qin-Lin* — 35

Hyperbaric oxygen in the management of skeletal muscle-compartment syndrome; *Michael B. Strauss, M.D., F.A.C.S., A.A.O.S., Diana A. Greenburg, R.N., M.S.N. and George B. Hart, M.D., F.A.C.S.* — 39

Hyperbaric oxygen therapy in the treatment of osteomyelitis; *M. Kawashima, H. Tamura and K. Takao* — 43

Intracranial Abscesses / Rationales for a therapeutic approach by hyperbaric oxygenation; *Lampl, L., Frey, G., Albert F. and Dietze T.* — 49

Neurological effects of diving and decompression sickness; *T. A. Anderson, R. G. Beran, C. W. Edmonds, R. D. Green and M. Hodgson* — 55

Changes of thromboxane A2 and prostacyclin in rabbits
suffering from decompression sickness; *J. Zhang, Supervisor:
Prof. G. T. Ni* — 65

The use and abuse of oxygen in Australian diving;
Carl Edmonds — 69

Effects of temperature on oxygen toxicity in rats at pressures
to 6 ATA.; *P. B. Bennett and K. E. Pinkerton* — 75

New developments in hyperbaric chambers;
Dr. -Ing. W. Lubitzsch — 85

The study of gas leakage test for saturation diving system with
air instead of helium; *Chen Hong-jun, Yu Hai-Quan, Cui Hai Liang,
Ren Xiao-Ling, Zheng Ru-Gen, Supervisor: Ni Guo-Tan* — 95

Air transportable emergency hyperbaric treatment systems /
Recent Australian experience; *I. Millar* — 99

Is transport of diving casualties under pressure worth it?;
Harry F. Oxer, M.A., F.F.A.R.A.C.S. — 103

Hyperbaric oxygen treatment for smoke inhalation in an
animal model; *Stewart, R. J., Yamaguchi, K. T., Knost, P. M.,
Noblett, K. L., Haworth, L. I. and O'Hara, V. S.* — 105

Carbon monoxide poisoning in New York City treatment
with hyperbaric oxygen; *E. Converse Pierce, II, M.D. and
William H. Bensky, P.A.* — 109

Cerebral thrombosis treated by hyperbaric oxygenation;
Wen-Ren Li, M.D. — 115

Does hyperbaric oxygen therapy prevent carbon
monoxide brain injury?; *Cohn, Gerald H., M.D., Cera, Peter J.,
M.D., Ehler, William, DVM., Hubbard, Eugene B., DVM, LTC, VC, Shiumazu, Takeshi, M.D., Sorts, R.W., DVM, Ph.D., Widden,
S.J., M.D., Ph.D. and Touhey, J. E., Col.* — 117

Hyperbaric oxygen therapy at 1.5 or 2.0 ATA as an
adjunct to the rehabilitation of stabilized stroke patients /
A controlled study; *A. Marroni, Data P. G. and Pilotti L.* — 123

Acute hydrogen sulphide poisoning treated with
hyperbaric oxygen; *Peng Hsu, M.D.* — 129

The ARMS experience of hyperbaric oxygen therapy
for multiple sclerosis; *D. J. D. Perrins, M.D., F.R.C.S.* — 137

The severe fat embolism treated by the combination therapy
using hyperbaric oxygen and conventional methods; *Hiroshi Yagi, Mitsuko Ohshima, Toshiro Yanai, Shozo Sadoshima and Hitoshi Fukui* — 141

Hyperbaric lung lavage in pulmonary alveolar proteinosis;
J. A. K. Peper, D.J. Bakker, C. M. Roos, J. J. Schreuder, W.W.A. Zuurmond and H. M. Jansen — 147

HBO treatment of gastric and duodenal ulcers; *Efuni S. N., Pogromov A. P., Egorov A. P. and Charayan L.V.* — 151

Hyperbaric oxygen at 2.0 or 2.5 ATA as an adjunct to levodopa
therapy of retinitis pigmentosa / A controlled study; *A. Marroni, De Iuliis G., Di Marzio L., De Sanctis G., Modugno G. and Data P. G.* — 157

Studies involving animal experiments to identify the action of
hyperbaric oxygen on the inner ear; *Pilgramm M., Mann W., Lohle E., Fischer B., Frey G., Lamm K. and Schmutz J.* — 163

Hyperbaric oxygen therapy in recent spinal cord injury;
John D. Yeo, A.O., M.B., M.S., D.P.R.M., F.R.A.C.S., F.A.C.R.M. — 169

The effect of pressure on the induction of ocular hyperuricosis;
William J. Ehler, Charles H. Bonney, Kwok-Wai Lam and John H. Cissik — 175

Hyperbaric oxygen in the therapy of aphonia associated with
chronic laryngitis; *Philip B. James Ph.D., M.F.O.M.* — 181

The effect of hyperbaric oxygenation on the function of
the adrenaline injured heart; *Demurov E. A., Koloskov Yu. B. and Smurova T. G.* — 185

A transportable recompression chamber system;
J. W. Pennefather — 189

Bronchial asthma treated by hyperbaric oxygen / A Report of 387 Cases; *Wen-Ren Li, M.D.* 193

Hyperbaric Medicine in China; *Wen-Ren Li, M.D.* 197

Hyperbaric oxygenation therapy for multiple sclerosis / A Report of 20 Cases; *Wen-Ren Li, M.D. and Zhou Xiu Zheng* 201

Myasthenia gravis treated by hyperbaric oxygenation / A Report of 40 Cases; *Wen-Ren Li, M.D., Li Jien Chen and Zhe Feng Jing* 205

The effects of high pressure of N_2 and He on neurotransmitter (dopamine) release from rat striatum; *R. B. Philp and M. L. Paul* 209

Hyperbaric oxygen and vasodilating therapy for idiopathic sudden hearing loss; *Goto F. Sasaki M. Kato K. Fujita T.* 215

Hyperbaric oxygen therapy for central nervous disorders / PET (positron on emission tomography) study; *Yasuharu Kitani, Katoko Miura, Yoshitaka Uchihashi and Tatsushi Fujita* 219

Change of breathing pattern at 3 ATA; *Tamaya, S., Makajima, I., Yamabayashi, H. and Ohta, Y.* 225

FOREWORD

On behalf of the Executive Committee of the Foundation for the International Congress on Hyperbaric Medicine, I am pleased to introduce the Proceedings of the IX International Congress on Hyperbaric Medicine published in a hard cover edition. This Congress was held in 1987 in Sydney, Australia, with President Ian P. Unsworth as a most gracious host. For the first time in the long history of the Congress the delegates assembled south of the equator. The meeting was most successful and a large number of persons attended from China and Japan. The Governors voted to convene in Amsterdam in 1990, which was a symbolic return to the birthplace of Clinical Hyperbaric Medicine on the occasion of the Tenth Congress. Through a special arrangement with Best Publishing Company, this edition completes the series of four books published with the same format which began with the Long Beach meeting in 1984. I wish to extend a special thank you to the publisher for their crucial role in making it possible at this time. The complete series of the four Proceedings documents the international field of scientific activity in Hyperbaric Medicine from 1984 to 1993. An additional thank you is extended to all of the authors whose diligent efforts make these publications possible.

Federick S. Cramer, M.D.
Secretariat
April, 1995

x

PROCEEDINGS OF THE IX INTERNATIONAL CONGRESS ON HYPERBARIC MEDICINE

These proceedings arise from the IX International Congress on Hyperbaric Medicine held in Sydney, Australia, in March 1987 at which a truly great representative group of hyperbaric specialists met. I was delighted at the broad spread of countries attending, illustrating the depth of Hyperbaric Medicine all around the globe. The friendliness of the delegates once again highlighted the maxim that "Medicine has no political boundaries."

What is not apparent from these bare publications is the enormous amount of discussion, planning and exchange of ideas carried on between all attendees on an informal level, in addition to formal committees, to decide the direction of Hyperbaric Medicine. There was a gratifying amount of accord in all areas. A major decision was to hold the Xth International Congress in The Netherlands in 1990.

I apologize for the delay between Congress and the publication of these Proceedings. I must ask for your indulgence but hope you will enjoy reading the papers presented in Sydney, on a wide range of hyperbaric and diving topics.

Ian P. Unsworth, M.D.,
President

Air and fat emboli in the lung and the brain

B. A. Hills

Department of Physiology
University of New England
Armidale N.S.W. Australia

Hyperbaric therapy with elevation of the inspired oxygen partial pressure is the treatment of choice for air embolism and decompression sickness. When a diver, caisson worker, aviator, astronaut or HBO chamber operator is decompressed beyond certain limits, he risks developing a wide range of symptoms which can be neatly fitted into six categories - five for aviators (1). One category is not necessarily an extension of the same insult causing another because each can be selected as the presenting symptoms by changing the conditions. Hence each category probably represents a different mechanism all of which are the subject of debate except for Category II where cerebral symptoms are almost certainly caused by arterial bubbles. The evidence is essentially that the same symptoms are observed following known air embolism caused iatrogenically or by pulmonary barotrauma.

EMBOLIC LIMITS

There has been much interest in the limits which the body can tolerate, the older surgical literature giving values for dogs of about 0.05 ml and 1.0 ml for air in the coronary and carotid arteries respectively, decreasing to as little as 0.025ml and 0.35ml for ischaemia in the myocardium and brain respectively (2,3). This is an order of magnitude of two less than the volume of a bolus which can be tolerated when injected into the venous system (4) - as reinforced by the advent of the Doppler meter and studies using it in the precordial position (5) to monitor the bubbles in total venous return.

PULMONARY BUBBLE TRAP

The above reasoning implies a very important role for the pulmonary circulation in trapping air in the venous system before it can reach the brain or myocardium where it could cause death if present in the volumes often detected by Doppler in the asymptomatic subject. By virtue of its location in the circulation, the lung is in a unique position to perform this function without which work in compressed air an hyperbaric therapy would be impossible.

My group has spent many years characterizing this important property of the pulmonary vasculature. When calibrated microbubbles are continuously infused into the venous system it is a big 'non-event' with nothing happening except a slight rise in alveolar P_{CO_2}. However, as soon as arterial bubbles are detected by Doppler, the whole scene changes (b) and the vital parameters show a dramatic decline in the general physiology of the animal. The point at which this occurs is determined by a remarkably well defined volume threshold of 0.35 ml/Kg. min in dogs (7).

DELAY IN ESCAPE

The interesting feature of bubble trapping by the lungs is that, when escape occurs, it does so after a delay of 10-90 minutes but, typically, about 20 minutes (6). Moreover bubble size is not of major importance. These facts indicate that bubbles are not retained by simple filtration, i.e. a sieving mechanism. This is consistent with the general lack of success in using filters to remove bubble from blood returning to the body from extracorporeal oxygenation circuits used in open-heart surgery (8) where both the membrane oxygenator and the pump have been implicated as the source of this very serious problem. Bubbles may be the cause of much of the morbidity and mortality associated with bypass surgery (8). Personally, I would like to see HBO therapy given post-operatively as a routine procedure so that its use in any specific case could not be misinterpreted to imply malpractice. My approach (9) to the problem has been to devise a new blood pump which we are developing here in Australia in which any bubbles are crushed by the application of extreme pressure (500-1,000 p.s.i.) for a few seconds. Since this pressure is applied isometrically, it avoids any injury to blood cells or platelets.

MECHANISM OF BUBBLE RETENTION

If the bubbles are not being sieved by the lung then they are probably being retained by capillarity. In the absence of anatomical shunts the vessels offering the greatest resistance to the displacement of blood by air needed for bubbles to traverse the lungs would be the smallest, i.e. the capillaries. Walder (10) performed a very important calculation in 1947 when he used the capillary equation ($P = 2y/r$) to calculate that, for a serum surface tension (y) of 50 dynes/cm, and capillary radius (r) of 5 mm, the displacement pressure (P) is 150 mmHg - which is far in excess of any attainable in the pulmonary artery and, hence, it was argued that air could not pass directly from venous to arterial blood through the lung unless there were shunts.

SURFACTANT MIGRATION

I realized (11) however, that this calculation makes numerous assumptions, including a contact angle of zero at the vessel wall and it ignores the effect of the trailing edge tending to propel the bubble forward. A third factor with an even greater effect in reducing the estimated value of AP is the use of a serum value for Y. Our studies (12) showed that surfactant from the lung can migrate into capillary blood if stasis is maintained by ligation or by embolization. This has many implications, my current interests pursuing the possible role of migrated surfactant in coating metastatic cells (13) temporarily arrested in pulmonary capillaries thereby reducing their potency to establish colonies - i.e. the "first organ effect" (14). Once again the lungs are in an unique location to monitor and control organ-to-organ traffic of emboli - whether metastatic cells or bubbles.

Returning to the bubble held by capillarity in the pulmonary capillary, migrated surfactant will have a strong affinity for the air interface by virtue of its amphipathic nature. Since this is the same surfactant which coats the alveolar surface, it is highly surface active with the capability of reducing surface tension to near zero (15). This would be disastrous since such a value would reduce AP to levels well below normal pulmonary arterial pressure when the lungs could never trap bubbles.

The mechanism by which surfactant exerts its role at the alveolar surface is a controversial issue (16) but one in which surfactant locating at an air-aqueous interface would probably reduce the surface tension to the equilibrium value of 25 dynes/cm or just below, i.e. down to 18 dynes/cm. When these values are used for Y, the pressure difference (A) for air to replace blood in the pulmonary capillary is reduced to 54-75 mm Hg which is now within the range of pulmonary arterial pressures which have been recorded following venous embolisation (18). Thus it is possible for bubbles to escape through the pulmonary capillaries but only after the migration of sufficient surfactant on to their surfaces. This could easily explain the characteristic time delay of 10-90 minutes in escape (6).

SURFACTANT

When bubbles are located in the pulmonary vasculature they have the ability to open the blood-lung barrier as demonstrated by Chryssanthou (19). Since they are chemically inert their action must be physical and it has been argued (16) that they could attract not only the migrating phospholipid but also the phospholipid in the pulmonary endothelial membrane which is also surface active. It is debatable whether the thermodynamic drive to locate at the bubble interface would be sufficient to dislodge the molecules comprising the phospholipid bilayer which is the basis of all membranes, pulmonary or otherwise (20). However, it could compete for a third lipid layer believed to be a monolayer or surfactant directly absorbed to the endothelium where it could effect control of permeability (21,16). By avoiding fixatives which remove surfactant, Ueda et al. (22) have recently produced a series of superb electron micrographs confirming direct absorption of surfactant onto pulmonary epithelium, while studies of the hydrophobic nature of the endothelium (23) are consistent with similar absorption to this membrane in some tissues.

BLOOD-BRAIN BARRIER

If bubbles have this ability to remove surface-active phospholipid from the endothelium, then it is most important to know what they do in the brain which is renowned for its tight junctions between endothelial cells which constitute the blood-brain barrier. Hence it is interesting to find several studies (19, 24, 25) indicating breakdown of the blood-drain by arterial air emboli. This is particularly important since the removal of the bubbles causing infraction by recompression is effected by their passage through the capillary bed, so that the treatment could be responsible for elutriating surface-active phospholipids from the endothelium and thus opening the blood-brain barrier.

EXPERIMENTAL

We have recently completed a series of runs using large (900 ± 100 gm) guinea pigs in which air or other embolic materials were injected into one carotid artery as 5ml of an ultrasonicated suspension in plasma from the same animal. After a period of 1,2,3, or 4 hours, Trypan blue was injected into the same carotid artery or the other and the animal sacrificed 15 minutes later and the brain excised. It was found that air emboli opened the blood-brain barrier in all cases, but it closed again between 2 and 3 hours after embolisation and was the same as the controls after 4 hours. Bubbles recovered from the brain were coated with surfactant but this could have been derived from blood.

MULTIPLE SCLEROSIS

In view of the controversial nature of the use of HBO in treating multiple sclerosis and the very interesting theory proposed by James (26) that MS is subacute fat embolism, it was decided to substitute depot fat or incomplete Freund's adjuvant (IFA) for air as the embolic material. The results were virtually the same as for air.

Since MS is a blood-brain barrier disease, these results not only confirm James' theory (26) but go on to indicate a very simple mechanism by which fat, or IFA in the EAE animal model can act. In a separate experiment, IFA was shown to be a superb solvent for the major phospholipids in membranes or absorbed to them. Thus fat or IFA could be simply dissolving the phospholipids, opening the blood-brain barrier, i.e. 'opening the door' for the next passing virus to enter the brain. No wonder the immunologists cannot agree upon the identity of the virus. This 'solvent' hypothesis (16) is also consistent with the wide use of adjuvants in agricultural research for promoting the immune response to vaccines.

We are now actively engaged in looking for the third layer on the endothelium which it is proposed limits permeability (21). This is contrary to the popular belief that all membranes are lipid bilayers on the basis that electron micrographs shown them as tramlines. However, before glutaraldehyde was adopted as an almost universal fixative, most e.m.s. depicted membranes as trilayers, e.g. the membrane around the optic nerve (30) and one relevant to MS since optic neuritis is often an early manifestation. Hence this study would strongly support James' claim (26) that multiple sclerosis is subacute fat embolism and, at the molecular level, would go to suggest a simple 'solvent' mechanism consistent with the classification of MS as a blood-brain barrier disease.

REFERENCES

1. Hills, B.A. (1982) Basic issues in prescribing preventive decompression. Undersea Biomed. Res.,9: 277-280.
2. Durant, T.M., Oppenheimer, M.J., Webster, M.R. and Long, J.(1949). Arterial air embolism. Amer. Heart J., 38: 481-500.
3. Kent, E.M. and Blades, B. (1942). Experimental observations upon certain intracranial complications of particular interest to the thoracic surgeon. J. Thorac. Surg., 11:434-445.
4. Durant, T.M., Long, J.M. and Oppenheimer, M.J. (1947). Pulmonary (venous) air embolism. Amer. Heart J., 33, 269-281.
5. Spencer, M.P. and Oyama, Y. (1971). Pulmonary capacity for dissipation of venous gas emboli. Aerospace Med., 42, 822-827.
6. Butler, B.D. and Hills, B.A. (1979). The lung as a filter for Microbubbles. J. Appl. Physiol.: Respir. Environ. Exercise Physiol., 47: 537-543.
7. Hills, B.A. and Butler, B.D. (1983). Air embolism: Further Basic Facts Relevant to the Placement of Central Venous Catheters and Doppler Monitors. Anesthesiology, 59: 163.
8. Bryan-Brown, C., Butler, B.D. and Hills, B.A. (1983). Air embolism, its sources, etiology, and prevention. In: Infusion Technology and Therapy. Technology Assessment Report 5-83, pp. 57-60. Washington: AAMI.
9. Hills, B.A. (1986). Blood Pumping Mechanism. U.S. Patent.
10. Walder, D.N. (1948). Serum surface tension and its relation to the decompression sickness of aviators. M.D. Thesis. University of Bristol, England. Journal of Physiology, 107:
11. Hills, B.A. (1977). Decompression Sickness. New York: Wiley.
12. Hills, B.A. and Butler, B.D. (1981). Migration of lung surfactant to pulmonary air emboli. In: Underwater Physiology VII. Ed. by Bachrach, A.J. and Matzen, M.M., pp. 741-752. Washington: Undersea Med. Soc.
13. Hills, B.A. (1984). Surfactant as a release agent opposing the adhesion of tumor cells in determining malignancy. Med. Hypoth. 14: 99-110.
14. Sherbert, G.V. (1982). The Biology of Tumour Malignancy. London: Academic.
15. Clements, J.A. (1957). Surface tension of lung extracts. Proc. Exper. Biol. Med., 95: 170-172.
16. Hills, B.A. (1987). The Biology of Surfactant. Cambridge: Cambridge U.P.

17. Bangham, A.D., Morley, C.J. and Phillips, M.C. (1979). The physical properties of an effective lung surfactant. Biochim. Biophys. Acta, 573: 552-556.
18. Josephson, S. (1970). Pulmonary air embolization in the dog. II Evidence and location of pulmonary vasoconstriction. Scand. J. Clin. Lab. Invest., 36: 113-123.
19. Chryssanthou, C., Spring, M. and Lipschitz, S. (1977). Blood-brain and blood-lung barrier alteration by dysbaric exposure. Undersea Biomed. Res., 4: 117-130.
20. Robertson, R.M. (1984). The Lively Membranes. Cambridge: Cambridge U.P.
21. Hills, B.A. (1985). Gastric mucosal barrier: stabilization of hydrophobic lining to the stomach by mucus., Amerc. J. Physiol. (Gastrointest. & Liver Physiol.), 244: G561-G568.
22. Ueda, S., Kawamura, K., Ishii, N., Matsumoto, S., Hayashi, K., Okayasu, M., Saito, M. and Sakurai, I. (1984). Ultrastructural studies on surface lining layer (SLL) of lungs: Part III of Nap. Med. Soc. Biol., Interface, 13: 76-88.
23. Sherman, I.A. (1981). Interfacial tension effects in the microvasculature. Micrvasc. Res., 22: 296-307.
24. Broman, T. (1947). Supravital analysis of disorders in the cerebral vascular permeability., II. Two cases of multiple sclerosis. Acta Psychiat. Scand. 46 (suppl.): 58-71.
25. Johansson, B. (1978). Blood-brain barrier dysfunction in experimental gas embolism. Underwater Physiology VI. Ed. by Schilling, C.W. and Beckett, M.W., pp.79-82. Washington: FASEB.
26. James, P.B. (1982). Evidence for subacute fat embolism as the cause of multiple sclerosis. Lancet, 13-2-82: 380-386.

Changes of rat spinal evoked potentials in acute decompression sickness

Xu Tie Supervisor: Prof. Ni Guo-Tan

Department of Naval Medicine, the Second Military Medical University, Shanghai, China

The acute decompression sickness (DCS) has been recognized for a long time. Many investigators work in order to find simple, exact and rapid method for monitoring DCS. Since 1981, Leitch and others have used the method of recording spinal evoked potentials (SEP) in monitoring spinal cord decompression sickness, developing an electrophysiological method for the diagnosis and qualification of the spinal cord DCS, evaluating the treatment.

But the previous works only be limited in the anesthetized dogs spinal cord DCS. The authors did not analyze the changes of different parts of SEP, and not point out their varies significance in monitoring spinal cord DCS.

The present work makes a model of rat acute decompression sickness, successively review the changes of SEP during the production, development and recompression treatment of acute DCS, and also review different changes of various parts of SEP. The significance of these changes was analyzed and discussed.

MATERIALS AND METHODS

Male SD rats, all conditioned and adult, weighting 250-350g were anesthetized with ip urethan (1000mg.kg^{-1}) and were given subcutaneous astropine (0.125mg) for reducing the trachea secretion. A catheter was placed in the trachea to maintain the animals natural ventilation.

The sciatic nerves, muscle and the vertebrae of T_{13} - L, were exposed, then finding the joint of T_{13} - L_1 and carefully eliminating adjacent muscle and subcutenous tissues. The rat was in prone position and it's vertebrae was fixed in a universal stereotaxic instrument (Chiang-Wan Model I-C).

Stimulating electrodes were pairs of stainless steel needles which hooked on the both side sciatic nerves. A silver ball-shaped single electrode 0.6mm in diameter was placed in the space between T_{13} - L_1. The reference electrode was put on the adjacent muscle of vertebrae. The gas bubbles were detected with a Doppler gas bubble detector (5MHz Model HYS-II).

The stimulus was delivered through a stimulus isolation (YGO-II) driven by a stimulus pulse generator (SBG-II). A stimulus of 3-5v with duration of O.1ms and rate of l.s^{-1} was given. The both side sciatic nerves were stimulated at the same time. The SEP signals from recording site went to a preamplifier (FZG-81) (gain 200) and filtered on a 100dHz bandpass. The output through the preamplifier was observed on a dual-beam oscilloscope (SBR-1) and filmed. Meantime, the signals (gain 40000) through the same preamplifier were recorded and printed by a microcomputer (TP-801A). The bubble sounds were recorded by cassette recorder (L-400).

The rats were divided into four groups: (I) the controls (n-5), in 2 hours at 101kpa, recording SEP at interval of 30 min. (II) the hyperbaric (n-5), in 2 hours at 1010kpa, recording SEP at interval of 30 min. (III) the safe decompression (n-10), were compressed to 1010kpa at a rate of 202kpa-min-1, 50 min at 1010kpa followed by decompressing rapidly to surface in 2 min. Ten rats were recompressed to 1010kpa when P_3, N_3 waves of SEP eliminated and when N_2 waves began to reduce or continuously reduced, the other twelve rats were recompressed to 1010kpa.

All animals in the chamber breathed air and were ventilated at intervals of 20 min. CO_2 in the chamber was maintained at 1% surface equivalent as measured by a gas chromatograph (Model-103) linked with a recording data processor (CDMC-II). The chamber temperature change was maintained in not exceeding ±2 °C.

After experiment, some animals spinal cords were taken out for eye observation and then fixed in 10% phosphate buffered formalin (4%wt/vol formaldehyde). The cord were cut into three segments, cervical, thoracic and lumber for light microscopic observation.

RESULT

GROUP I: the SEP peak latency, spread and amplitude did not any changes. GROUP II: the SEP peak latency and spread did not changes, amplitude had some decreasing, but not significant. GROUP III: the parameters of SEP were not significantly changed. GROUP IV: in 2-10 min. after rapid decompression all animals had grade III gas bubble sound (Spencer's) and "chokes" sign (DCS appeared). P_3, N_3 waves amplitude rapidly reduced and lost ($P<0.05$); N_2 waves amplitude showed some reducing. At this moment, recompression was given to ten animals. After 4-30 min of recompression (1010kpa), P_3, N_3 and N_2 waves recovered to normal level. Their amplitudes had significant differences compared with those during DCS ($P<0.05$) and no significant changes compared with those of pre-decompression. Bubble sound and "chokes" sign also eliminated (seeing Fig.1 CONTROL = SEP of 101kpa; H=SEP of 1010kpa; DCS = 4 min after decompression, animal had grade III gas bubble sound and "chokes" sign, P_3, N_3 disappeared and N_2 reduced; C=20 min after recompression (1010kpa), amplitude of P_3, N_3 and N_2 waves had recovered to normal level).

When N_2 continuously decreased or it's wave peak paralleled N1 wave peak, twelve animals were recompressed. Under these circumstances the animals were close to death, recompression could not obtain any positive result. At last N_2 wave lost but P_1, N_1 and P_2 waves no changes, but followed

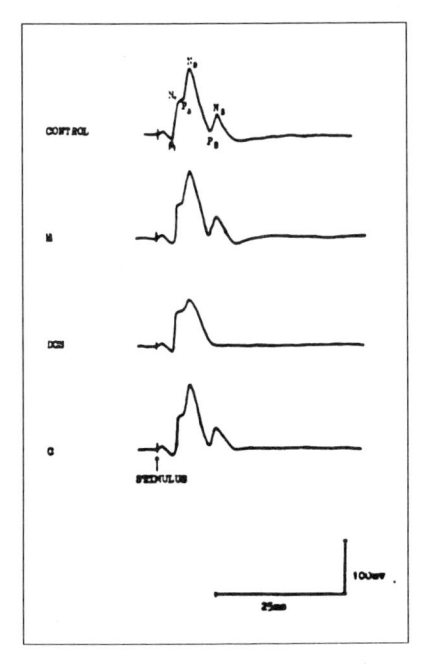

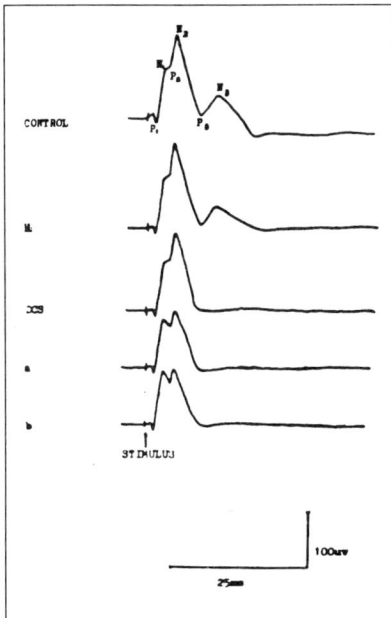

Figure 1.

Figure 2.

the prolongation of postmortal duration, these waves also could not be evoked. The values of these waves had no significant difference compared with the pre-decompression. (seeing Fig.2: CONTROL = SEP OF 101kpa; H = SEP of 1010kpa; DCS = 6 min after decompression the animal had grade III gas bubble sound and "chokes" sign. P_3, N_3 eliminated and N_2 reduced; a=8 min after decompression, N_2 went on reducing, began to recompress; b=during recompression, N_2 continuously reduced, the animal's respiration ceased).

Anatomical examination showed that no gas bubbles were found in the lung, heart, vertebrae tube and spinal cord vessels of Group I,II,III and animals that effected to respond to recompression. Many gas bubbles were widely seen in the animals that failed to respond to recompression.

Light microscopic observations showed that red cell emboli in the white matter, asmotic hemorrhage in the grey matter and gas bubbles in the spinal cord posterior artery of the animals which failed to respond to recompression.

DISCUSSION

Rat spinal cord evoked potentials composed of rapid waves (early parts, P_1, N_1, P_2) and slow waves (late parts, N_2, P_3, N_3). Rapid waves come from primary afferent volley of peripheral nerves and slow waves come from synthesis response of synaptic and pro-synaptic electric activities in spinal cord. The latter is more dependent on energy and oxygen supply.

In acute decompression sickness, the autochthonous gas bubbles in various locations may cause spinal cord vessels aeroembolism, the lung aeroembolism which cause secondary diffusion fails, and the heart-failed which cause tissue ischemia. These pathophysiological changes interrupt the supports of energy and oxygen to the spinal cord synaptic transmission. So, when DCS appears, slow waves produce response at first. If the recompression may be timely put into effect, the gas bubbles in the body may be eliminated so that the blood perfusion recovers, and the SEP can return to normal level and DCS can also disappear. If the recompression is given too late, N_2 continuously reduces or loses, the recompression can scarcely achieve any effective result, and the animals are close to death. The rapid waves often do not have significant changes at a shorter time after animals death, because peripheral nerve conduction needs lesser energy and oxygen than synaptic transmission.

In Group II (the hyperbaric), the SEP parameters did not change in 2 hours, which showed that effects of high pressure air on SEP is scarce. This result is coincident with Leitch's.

The experimental results suggest that the SEP may be used to monitor acute decompression sickness; the SEP has a remarkable changes which successively occurs from slow waves to rapid waves; the reflect of slow waves to DCS is susceptible compared with rapid waves, depending on the alterations of SEP amplitude to monitor the process of occurrence, development and recovery of acute DCS; as soon as the changes of slow waves, especially P_3, N_3 waves, appear, acute DCS must be seriously paid attention to and at this moment recompression may return the SEP to normal, DCS may be eliminated; when rapid waves show changes, the animal is generally in an irreversible condition.

Appearance and disappearance of gas bubble sound is consistent with loss and recovery of slow waves, they have a linear relationship.

Control of HPNS with Trimix 5 (5% N_2/He/O_2) to 600 m

Peter B. Bennett, Richard D. Vann, Henry Schafstall, J. Holthaus and W. Schnegelsberg

F.G. Hall Laboratory, Duke Medical Center
Durham, North Carolina, USA
and GKSS/GUSI
Geesthacht, Federal Republic of Germany

INTRODUCTION

Although Hannes Keller made a brief open sea dive to 300 m in the early sixties, it is only seventeen years ago in 1969 that a full scale simulated saturation dive to 300 m was made collaboratively by the U.S. Navy and the F.G. Hall Laboratory at Duke (1). Since then deep diving research has continued at many international centers to investigate the problems and control of High Pressure Nervous Syndrome (HPNS) to permit successful ultra deep diving (2) and solve the difficulties of safe decompression from great depths (3). In 1981 this research culminated at Duke during the 4 deep Atlantis research dives (4), in a record simulated research dive by 3 men at the F.G. Hall Laboratory to 686 m (2250 ft) (5).

These dives were designed to compare the effectiveness in controlling the many signs and symptoms of HPNS such as tremors, nausea, dizziness, vomiting, increased EEG theta (6-8 Hz) activity and performance decrements to 650 and 686 m by variation of the rate of compression or addition of 5 or 10% nitrogen to the helium-oxygen normally used in deep diving. An intensive series of pulmonary, psychometric, hematologic and other tests were made (4,5). In addition, much knowledge was gained on decompression from such great depths utilizing various continuous rates of decompression dependent on the oxygen partial pressure and the depth.

The least signs and symptoms of HPNS and decrement in performance from a cognitive and psychomotor view, as shown in Figs. 1 and 2 respectively, were obtained by use of Trimax 5, i.e. 5% nitrogen in heliox. This was combined with a slow exponential rate of compression and the regular use of stages at which several hours were spent without compression to permit adaptation to the pressure (4,5).

The GKSS Research Center, Geesthacht GmbH, near Hamburg conducts pre-industrial research and development on behalf of the Federal Republic of Germany in the fields of environmental protection, material technology and underwater technology. Underwater research and development objectives are aimed at finding technical solutions for the safe and efficient performance of underwater work including installation, maintenance and repair. They include necessary diving techniques, underwater testing, safety of underwater work and training of underwater specialists.

Early efforts in this regard started over 12 years ago with the operation of the open sea habitat "HELGOLAND" and associated diving equipment. In 1980-83 a very large ocean simulator system was installed by Draeger, Lubeck. Designed by GKSS in cooperation with industry and universities, the GKSS Underwater Simulator Plant (GUSI) is one of the largest and most sophisticated systems in the world today. Manned diving tests are possible to a simulated salt water depth of 600 m and unmanned tests down to 2200 m. The largest pressure chamber is 3.5 m internal diameter and 12.7 m long. It can be filled with salt water and is connected by a vertical chamber to two living chambers. In addition the temperature can be varied from 0-32°C (Fig. 3).

As a consequence of the extensive experience of the Duke F.G. Hall Laboratory staff in deep saturation diving, they were contacted at an early stage in the operation of the German facilities and in the training of GUSI staff in saturation diving techniques and to produce safe operational procedures to 600 m.

GUSI is designed for technical work at pressure and not primarily for medical research and therefore needed conservative compression and decompression schedules to permit the divers to reach maximum depth and be able to start welding or other technical research work as soon as possible and to return to the surface safely. It was important also that there be no long lasting deleterious effects from such exposures.

METHODS

It was decided that for optimal relief from the signs and symptoms of HPNS, and without the problems of nitrogen narcosis, compression would be with TRIMIX 5 (i.e. 5% nitrogen, O.5 bar oxygen and remainder helium) throughout. Indeed the same gas mixture was chosen for all GUSI dives including the decompression.

Evolving from the Duke 'Atlantis' experience above, a compression profile was selected to 600 m (Table 1). A series of dives were then planned, using this profile, from 1983 to 1986 which would gradually work down to the maximum operating depth of 600 m contingent upon there being no deleterious HPNS effects in the divers (Table 2).

The decompression procedures are shown in Table 3 and are based on evaluation of 1055 helium-oxygen man-decompressions and 189 nitrogen-oxygen-man-decompressions (3) and the equation $R = K*PIO_2$, where R is measured in m/hr or fsw/hr, PIO_2 is in ATM (or bars), and the proportionality constant is in m/ATM or fph/ATM. The data suggested that it is necessary to reduce the value of K as the depth of dive increases. The schedules generated from the estimated K values are with O.5 bar oxygen to a depth of 14 m, after which the oxygen is held at O.21 bar until surfacing.

From 1983 to September 1986 an extensive series of 8 major studies with 14 deep dives between 300 m - 600 m were made using 13 German, English, French and American divers and involving 1,341 man days of saturation in 50 man-dives (Table 2). These divers were not especially selected and the majority had not experience of such deep saturation diving.

In most cases while the first group of four divers were decompressing a second group were compressed to meet them for saturation at a shallower depth and then all divers decompressed together.

Extensive clinical and psychological testing of the divers was made annually leading to an offshore diving medical fitness certificate according to the UK/Norway Offshore Diving Standards. This included initial clinical psychological evaluations by the experienced DFVLR aerospace group at Hamburg, chest and long bone x-rays and a T_C 99 m per technetate scan every two years plus full head EEG and neurological evaluation (6). Immediately before and after every dive a further physical evaluation was made by usually two physicians.

During the dive, monopolar EEG was recorded from the occipital region with eyes open and shut and fast fourier frequency analysis was provided. Similarly a neurological examination was made on arrival at maximum depth and on arrival at the second work depth during decompression.

Daily check-off sheets were provided to identify any HPNS, nitrogen narcosis or other adverse signs or symptoms and included answers for presence of dreams, degree of sleep and location of aches or pains on a manikin diagram. This was accompanied by regular verbal questioning of the divers.

Muscle strength was tested by a hand held dynamometer which recorded peak grip and strength over a fixed time of 1 min. A two hour clinical psychological test package of vigilance and memory especially, were made by Dr. Goeters of DFVLR before the dives to 500 and 600 m and at depth and on return to the surface. These consisted of four tests. Test KBT (author Kirsch) required steady and coordinated use of perception speed, memory capability and calculating ability. Test MEK (author Kirsch) measured the memory capacity for visual information. Test UZA (author Winke) measured the memory capacity for auditory perception and the CLE test (author Witt) measured the memory capacity for acoustically transmitted information.

In addition to this, especially in the 600 m dive, Dr. Richard Moon collected venous blood to study platelet and other changes and also urine volume and electrolytes were recorded. Body weight was recorded through the dives.

A practical test of the efficiency of the procedures was the ability of the divers to go to work as required after arrival at depth and carry out necessary chamber function and breathing apparatus tests as well as various forms of welding while wearing breathing apparatus for a full workday.

RESULTS

The results indicated little or no HPNS during compressions and hardly any compression arthralgia. The divers were fit on arrival and functionally normal with no indications of nausea, visible tremors, or undue fatigue. At 500 m in GUSI 7, one diver did vomit immediately after breakfast a day after compression but he did then develop a viral infection with increased temperature which resulted in him being taken off work. At 450 m in GUSI 5 two French divers made a certification weld of a 36 inch steel pipe and finished ahead of schedule affirming that the depth felt less than 100 m.

The performance tests showed little change to 500 m. Only the KBT test of perception speed, memory and calculating capability showed any significant decrements at 500 m and at the 278 m depths although the decrement was less (Table 4) at 278 m.

At 600 m the performance decrement was more general, especially in the tasks requiring memory. Thus again the KBT test of perceptions speed memory and calculating ability was significantly decreased (Table 5) but in addition the CLE test of memory capacity and auditory information was also significantly lower (Table 6). However, this was not noticed in the ability of the divers to function at their welding and chamber function tests although they remarked that extra concentration was required. They appeared apparently normal with no adverse remarks on their check lists except for obligate mouth breathing being required at depths in excess of 450 m.

The EEG activity was remarkably free of HPNS related theta activity (6-8 Hz) in all divers, even during the 600 m dive (Fig. 3). The particular subject shown in Fig. 3 was also a subject in the Atlantis dives which unlike this dive did produce increased theta activity and HPNS with the faster compressions. Of special interest in the EEG was the abolition or reduction of the alpha activity (Fig. 4). Again in this diver no theta activity is seen but the large normal alpha activity (8-13 Hz) initiated with eyes closed which usually is markedly reduced or blocked by opening the eyes, was eliminated by the pressure itself from 360 m to 600 m.

Body weight declined especially in the 600 m dive with some subjects being more susceptible than others. This weight loss which continued into decompression was partially reestablished closer to the surface by encouraging drinking formula fluids (Table 7) and was fully restored after return to surface. From evidence to be presented elsewhere it is clear the the weight loss is primarily due to dehydration and studies were made of an increase in atrial matriuretic peptide (h.ANP) in plasma as the possible cause.

Dynamometer tests at 500-600 m showed an average reduction of between -3% to -13% in peak strength with little change in the duration strength test.

During the 50 man dives three decompression incidents are of note. During GUSI 7 one of the divers at 7.8 m complained of difficulty in sleeping. He was a diver from the shallower 300 m saturation and some twenty minutes after announcing this problem he reported left knee pain. He was given 3 twenty minute periods of pure oxygen to breathe and the pain resolved without recompression. After 6 hr the decompression was continued on the original schedule.

Similarly in GUSI 8 one of the 600 m divers awoke at 40 m complaining of constant left knee pain for twenty minutes. When it reappeared some hours later for the same time the physician ordered three 20 min oxygen breathing cycles. Two days later recurring "niggles" of the right knee also resulted in a further three cycles of breathing treatment gas.

Finally another of the 600 m divers presented a neurological deficit in his right foot during the post dive examination on surfacing with "foot drop", muscular weakness and sensory deficit on both sides of the foot. He was treated with recompression and oxygen and saturated at 18 m for 24 hrs and recovered. It is pertinent that this diver had some evidence of foot drop in his pre-dive physical and so it would seem the decompression from 360 m singled out this particular site of earlier injury.

DISCUSSION AND CONCLUSION

This is a unique number of 14 very deep dives made in a relatively short time of 2-3 years. Trimix 5 (nitrogen 5%/O_2) 0.5 bar/helium remainder) when combined with the Duke slow exponential compression profile with long stages seems to permit divers to reach 600 m or lesser depths with remarkably little or not signs and symptoms of HPNS and able to work effectively at welding or other tasks. Importantly, the presence of nitrogen in the breathing gas also does not appear to affect the integrity of the weld.

The divers showed no post diving effects other than the usual cardiorespiratory debilitation for a week or so as a result of the confinement, lack of exercise, sunshine and weight loss.

The performance tests indicated decrements at only the 500 and 600 m depths and yet the divers' activity at the welding and other tasks did not appear to be impaired. However, the results do indicate that performance efficiency can be expected to start to fall off at depths much in excess of 600 m. A part of this could well be due to the 5% nitrogen but it is felt that this is the price to be paid for control of the unpleasant signs and symptoms of HPNS which is the alternative and would be likely to be more incapacitating in some cases. Similar decrements were reported in Atlantis III (7) in 3 divers at 686 m breathing 10% nitrogen in heliox. This data also showed that divers can continue to function at such extreme depths but changes became apparent in tasks requiring rapid problem solving abilities or extended long term memory. Extensive training could help to reduce these factors and may be important to the divers ability to react correctly in a sudden emergency.

The reduction or abolition of the alpha activity in the EEG at the greater depths is also an indication that physiological changes are occurring although there is no physical sign at this depth. The lack of HPNS induced theta activity is most encouraging. On the other hand the loss of alpha activity may be due to a generalized reduction in electrical activity of the brain which has been reported in previous deep dives or an electrical alerting of the brain.

The linear decompression profiles were of necessity very long. Indeed it seems that the deeper the dive the slower must be the decompression. Yet even with rates as slow a O.75 m/hour (2.5 ft/hr) some signs and symptoms of decompression sickness were seen close to or at the surface, and this in the two 600 m divers even though they had spent over two days saturated during the decompression at 360 m. It might therefore be assumed that some gas from the 600 m to 360 m part of the dive still remained in the divers as the normal rate for a decompression from 360 m alone would be much faster at 3.3 ft/hr which was done by many of the divers without any adverse effect (Table 3).

Thus the diver in GUSI 7 who complained of decompression sickness had made three previous decompressions from the 300 m depth, to which the diver had been exposed, at decompression rates much faster and with no effect.

The decompressions are singularly difficult due to their length and yet still causing decompression sickness. The length is a major problem as it involves many weeks for the diver living in a small space like an astronaut with limited exercise and social interaction and in an environment of boredom to which too little attention has been paid in the past.

Nevertheless these dives are a prominent milestone in the attempts to permit divers to live and work at greater depths and indicate that sixteen years after the first dive to 300 m, man now can work effectively, using the techniques described, at 600 m.

ACKNOWLEDGEMENT

This work represents the efforts of large teams of support staff from the GKSS GUSI and Duke University F.G. Hall Laboratory including physicians, engineers, chamber supervisors, chamber operators, technicians and many more who worked night and day for months at a time and without which the dives could not have been done. Above all, we wish to thank the divers themselves who remained saturated inside the pressure chambers for times as long as 43 days. The undoubted success of these dives is a pertinent reward for their dedication and hard work.

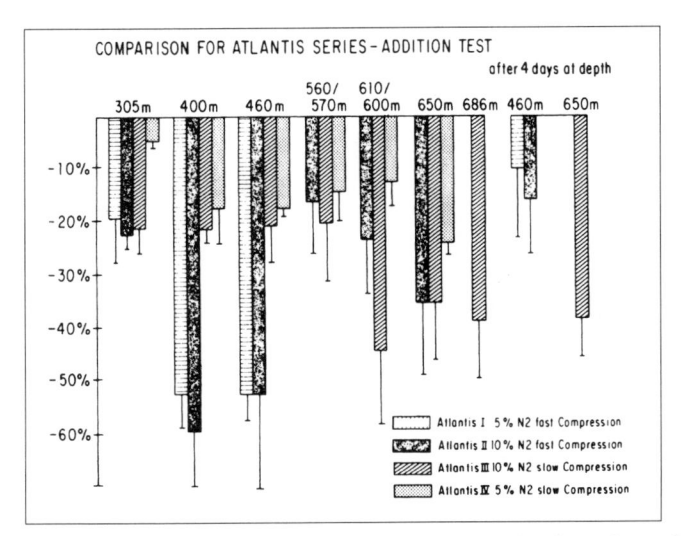

Figure 1. Comparison of the mean percentage decrement of 3 divers for each of the dives Atlantis I, II, III and IV at the arithmetic test involving memory and cognition. The larger decrements at 400 and 600 m for I and II due to fast compression is clear as is the increasing decrement for dives greater than 500 m for dives II and III but the considerable benefit in Atlantis IV of 5% nitrogen and slow compression (4).

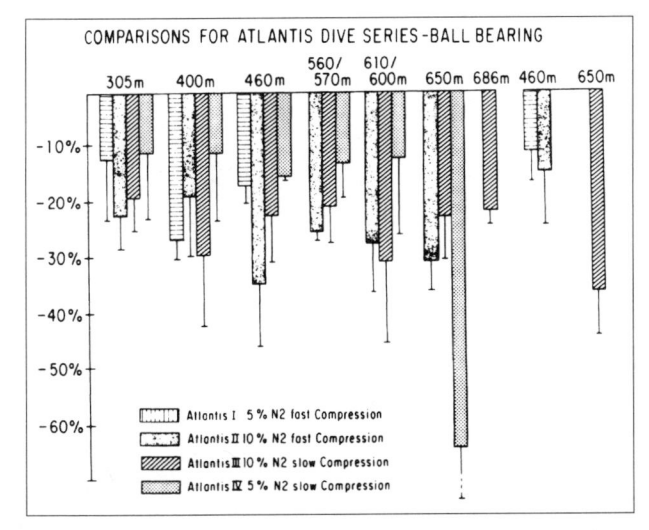

Figure 2. Comparison of the mean percentage decrement of 3 divers for each of the dives Atlantis I, II, III and IV at the ball bearing test of fine motor dexterity. Except for 650 m the lowest nitrogen (5%) and slow rate of compression of the Atlantis IV indicate the least psychomotor decrement.

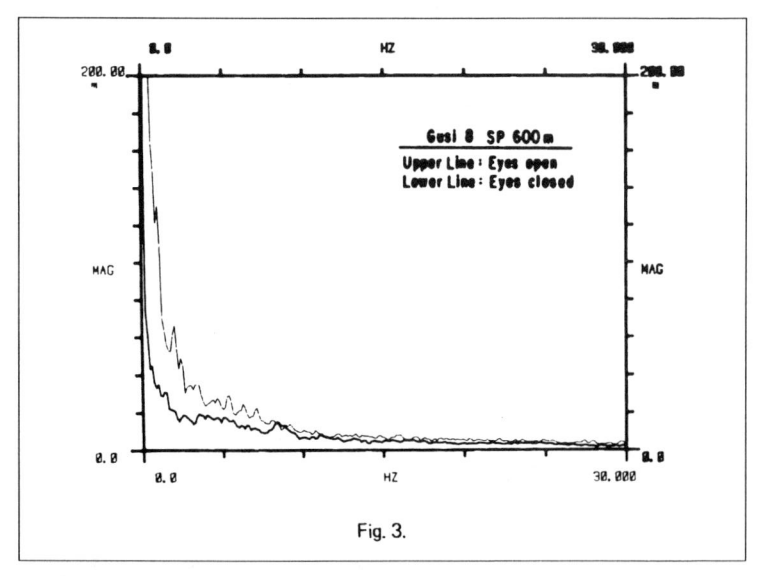

Figure 3. Fast Fourier Frequency analysis of the occipital EEG of a diver at 600 m. Upper line eyes open, bottom eyes closed. No increase in slow wave activity seen. The other two subjects were the same.

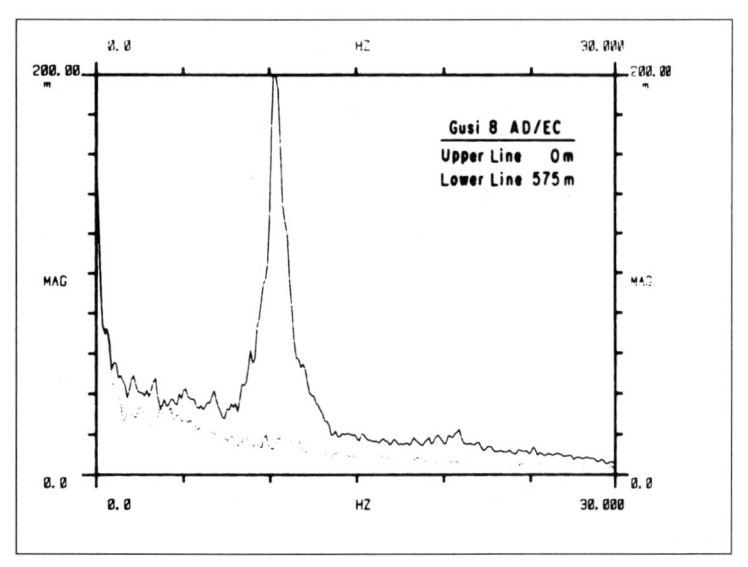

Figure 4. Fast Fourier Frequency analysis of occipital EEG of a diver with eyes closed at surface predive (upper line). It may be seen that the alpha frequency at 8-13 Hz has disappeared at 575 m.

Table 1. Duke/GUSI Compression Profile to 600 m with Trimix 5 (N_2 5%/0.5 bar O_2/He rest)

Travel 0 m - 180 m	= 5 m/min (36 min)
Stop at 180 m	= 2 hrs
Travel 180 m - 240 m	= 3 m/min (20 mins)
Stop at 240 m	= 6 hrs
Travel 240 m - 300 m	= 1.5 m/min (40 mins)
Stop at 300 m	= 2 hrs
Travel 300 m - 350 m	= 0.5 m/min (1 hr 40 mins)
Stop at 350 m	= 9 hrs
Travel 350 m - 400 m	= 0.25 m/min (3 hr 20 min)
Stop at 400 m	= 2 hrs
Travel 400 m - 430 m	= 0.125 m/min (4 hrs)
Stop at 430 m	= 2 hrs
Travel 430 m - 460 m	= 0.125 m/min (4 hrs)
Stop at 460 m	= 12 hrs
Travel 460 m - 490 m	= 0.100 m/min (5 hrs)
Stop at 490 m	= 2 hrs
Travel 490 m - 520 m	= 0.100 m/min (6 hr 40 min)
Stop at 520 m	= 13 hrs
Travel 520 m - 550 m	= 0.075 m/min (6 hr 40 min)
Stop at 550 m	= 13 hrs
Travel 550 m - 575 m	= 0.05 m/min (8 hr 20 min)
Stop at 575 m	= 16 hrs
Travel 575 m - 600 m	= 0.05 m/min (8 hr 20 min)

Table 2. GUSI/Duke Dive 1983-1986

DIVES	DATE	DIVE DAYS	NO. OF DIVERS	MAN DIVES
GUSI 1 125/300/150 m	23 Nov 1983 to 16 Dec 1983	24	4	96
GUSI 2 150 m	12 March 1984 to 21 March 1984	10	3	29
GUSI 3 300/150 m	7 May 1984 to 27 May 1984	21	3 (300 m) 3 (150 m)	86
GUSI 4 400/200 m	2 Sept 1984 to 29 Sept 1984	28	3 (400 m) 3 (200 m)	135
GUSI 5 450/265 m	14 Nov 1984 to 14 Dec 1984	32	4 (450 m) 4 (265 m)	173
GUSI 6 450/265 m	23 April 1985 to 24 May 1985	35	4 (450 m) 4 (265 m)	198
GUSI 7 500/450/300 m	6 Nov 1985 to 10 Dec 1985	35	4 (500 m) - (450 m) 4 (300 m)	280
GUSI 8 600/360 m	20 March 1986 to 1 May 1986	43	4 (600 m) 4 (360 m)	344
TOTALS		224	50	1341

Table 3. Provisional Duke Saturation Decompression Schedules (MSW)

Oxygen   - 0.5 ATM partial pressure deeper than 14 msw
               - 21% from 14 msw to surface
Nitrogen   - Not more than 5% deeper than 15 msw
               - Not more than 0.79 ATM partial pressure at less than 150 msw
Helium   - Balance

SATURATION DEPTH, MSW	KE, FPH/ATM	UNTIL 14 MSW	14 TO 9 MSW	9 TO 6 MSW	6 TO 3 MSW	3 TO 0 MSW	DAY	HR
0 - 30	12.0	17	21	25	30	40	0	22
30 - 60	11.0	18	23	27	33	43	1	17
60 - 90	10.0	20	25	30	36	47	2	18
90 - 120	9.5	21	26	31	38	50	3	18
120 - 150	9.0	22	28	33	40	53	4	21
150 - 180	8.5	24	29	35	43	56	6	7
180 - 210	8.5	24	29	35	43	56	7	7
210 - 240	8.0	25	31	37	45	59	8	15
240 - 270	8.0	25	31	37	45	59	9	16
270 - 300	7.5	27	33	39	48	63	11	13
300 - 330	7.5	27	33	39	48	63	12	16
330 - 360	7.0	29	36	42	52	67	14	20
360 - 390	7.0	29	36	42	52	67	16	1
390 - 410	6.5	31	38	45	56	73	18	0
410 - 450	6.5	31	38	45	56	73	19	18
450 - 480	6.0	33	41	49	60	79	22	10
480 - 510	6.0	33	41	49	60	79	23	19
510 - 540	5.5	36	45	54	66	86	27	11
540 - 570	5.5	36	45	54	66	86	28	23
570 - 600	5.0	40	50	59	72	94	33	20
600 - 630	4.5	44	55	65	80	105	39	1
630 - 686	4.0	50	62	73	90	118	48	6

RATE OF ASCENT, MIN/(.5 MSW); DECOMPRESSION TIME

Table 4. GKSS/DFVLP Test KBT (Goeters/Kirsch) perception speed, memory, calculation

	MEAN	SEM	T TEST
Pre-Dive	79.25	±26.17	—
500 m	47.00*	±23.19	1%
278 m	70.50	±27.04	1%
Post-Dive	97.00	±28.52	—

Table 5. GKSS/DFVLR Test KBT (Goeters/Kirsch) perception speed, memory, calculation

	MEAN	SEM	T TEST
Pre-Dive	94.33	±36.35	—
600 m	59.33	±34.39	5%
510 m	65.67	±40.99	5%
Post-Dive	90.66	±41.47	—

Table 6. GKSS/DFVLR Test CLE (Goeters/Witt) memory capacity and auditory information

	MEAN	SEM	T TEST
Pre-Dive	207.67	±11.69	—
600 m	151.33	±30.09	1%
510 m	170.67	±34.96	—
Post-Dive	188.33	±29.53	—

Table 7. Body weights (KG) during 600 M dive

	S1	S2	S3	S4	MEAN
CONTROL	95	81	76.5	93	86.4
599 m	92.3	79.1	74	88	83.4
474 m	91	76.8	72.8	86	82.0
360 m	89.8	75.7	72.1	84.7	80.4
259 m	89.1	76.7	73.0	84.5	80.8
134 m	88.8	75.3	73.3	84.3	80.4
Surface	90.0	77.5	73.8	84.0	81.3

REFERENCES

1. Summit JK, Kelly JS, Heron JM, Saltzman, HA. 1000 ft helium saturation exposure. In: Lambertson, CJ ed. Proc. 4th symposium underwater physiology. New York; Academic Press. 1971: 519-527.
2. Bennett PB. The high pressure nervous syndrome in man. In: Bennett PB and Elliott DH, eds. The physiology and medicine of diving. San Pedro, CA; Best Publishers. 1982: 262-296.
3. Vann RD. Decompression from saturation diving. In: Rosser DR, ed. Proceedings 3rd annual canadian ocean technology conference. Toronto; Underwater Canada. 1984: 175-186.
4. Bennett PB, McLeod M. Probing the limits of human deep diving. Phil Trans R Soc Lond B 1984; 304: 105-117.
5. Bennett PB, Coggin R, McLeod M. Effect of compression rate on use of trimix to ameliorate HPNS in man to 686 m (2250 ft). Undersea Biomed Res 1982; 9:335-351.
6. Holthaus J, Bennett PB. Medical cover and diver monitoring for very deep saturation working dives at GUSI. GKSS-Forschungszentrum, Geesthacht GmbH 1985 Report No 85/E/57.
7. Logue PE, Schmitt FA, Rogers HE, Strong GB. Cognitive and emotional changes during a simulated 686 meters.deep dive.

Change in lung diffusion capacity (LDC) during acute decompression sickness (DCS) in awake rabbits

Jiang Jian-Yong, Supervisor: Prof. Ni Guo-Tan

Department of Naval Medicine, the Second Military Medical University, Shanghai, China

The lung, by virtue of its central location within the circulation, is a major target organ for bubble emboli liberated in venous blood during decompression. Respiratory DCS, known to divers as the 'chokes', is probably the result of pulmonary bubble embolism (PBE). It has been postulated that the presence of significant numbers of venous gas emboli (VGE) interfere with inert gas elimination and thus are involved in the pathogenesis of DCS. The pulmonary hypertension, systemic hypotension, hemoconcentration and hypoxemia are typical responses to decompression. To date neither the effect of severe decompression associated with PBE on pulmonary gas exchange on the pathogenesis of hypoxemia in acute DCS has been described completely. The purpose of this study was to examine the hypothesis that alterations in LDC due to PBE plays an important role in the pathogenesis of hypoxemia in acute DCS.

METHODS

General: Thirty-four male rabbits (new Zealand) weighing 2.2±2.25 kg were divided into three groups: (A) the rapid decompression (N-18), 30 min at 808 Kpa followed by decompression in 3 min. (B) the safe decompression (N-8), 30 min at 808 Kpa followed by stage decompression in 45 min. (C) the controls (N-8), only staying in the chamber at 101 Kpa for 33 min. The animals were turned to the supine position, restrained and intubated following local anaesthesia with 1% novocaine, then left undisturbed for 30 min before the experiments began.

Doppler bubble detection: Using a 5MHz Model HYS-II Doppler bubble detector (Naval Medical Research Institute, Shanghai, China), VGE due to decompression was detected. The exact position of the point yielding the best signal of the pulmonary artery was marked on the animal's chest insuring reproducible sensorplacement. For the precordial signals, Spence's 0-4 scale for estimating bubble quantities was adopted.

Measurement of LDC for carbon monoxide (LDCco): The standard single-breath Method was modified in order to be performed on animals.

Briefly, when the rabbit breathed out to functional residual volume, 30 ml the test gas (N_2 76.20%, O_2 20.01%, He 3.45%, CO 0.34%) was infused into its lung through the endotracheal tube, held the breath for 10s then the gas was withdrawn slowly; after the withdrawal of 10 ml, a sample of 2 ml of alveolar gas was collected for analysis. The gas was analyzed with a gas chromatograph Model 103 (Analysis Instrument Inc. Shanghai, China) associated with a Model CDCM-II Recording Data Processor (Comput Technique Institute, Shanghai, China).

Blood gas measurement: Partial Pressures of O_2 (PaO_2), CO_2 ($Paco_2$), the percentage of oxygen saturation ($O_2SAT\%$), the oxygen content (O_2CT Vol%), K_+ of serum, the concentration of hemoglobin (Hb g%) and pH were measured on samples drawn from the femoral artery with the aid of an automatic system for blood gas analysis Model ABL-4 (Radio Comp, Denmark).

Experimental protocol: Experimental rabbits were prepared as previously described. Measurements of Doppler recordings, LDCco were performed 15 min pre-exposure to hyperbaric or control condition and postexposure. In six rabbits of Group A, blood gas analyses and Doppler detection were simultaneously made at 10 min prior to exposure and at 10, 20, 30, 45, and 60 min after the decompression unless the animals died. Except the six rabbits, all animals were removed from restraint in order for us to observe the presence of any intravenous injection of KC1. Autopsy was immediately performed. The lungs were excised and fixed for light microscopic examination.

Statistics: We made all comparison by paired t tests or by analysis of variance. We accepted P<0.05 as indicating statistical significance. The correlations were tested by using Spearman's rank correlation method.

RESULTS

In Group A, all animals developed bends, dyspnea and paraplegia. Ten of them died earlier than 45 min postdive with Doppler signals ranging from 2-4 grads and others (N-8) survived for more than 45 min after back to surface with 1-3 grade of Doppler signals. They respectively suffered from severe and mild DCS. The rabbits of Group B and C showed neither signs of DCS nor more than 1 grade of Doppler signals. Table 1 shows the results of the studies of LDCco. A statistically significant difference in LDCco occurred in Group A (paired t test, P<0.01). There was no significant difference in either in Group B or in Group C. A surprising finding was that there is a significant correlation between the decrease in LDCco and the grade of Doppler bubble signals (r-P.767, P<0.01).

A1 including the animals with severe DCS; A2 including the animals with mild DCS; n, number of rabbits. Values are group averages (SD);
*Significant difference from base-line by paired t test or by F test as P<0.05.

Table 1. LDCco in various experimental groups

Group	n	(LDCco(mmolmin^{-1}Kpa$_1$ Kg^{-1}) preexposure (15 min)	postexposure 15 min	Bubble grade.
A	18	0.0739(0.0153)	0.0395(0.0196)*	1-4
A1	10	0.0765(0.0107)	0.0282(0.0140)*	2-4
A2	8	0.0705(0.0199)	0.0537(0.0163)*	1-3
B	8	0.0648(0.0064)	0.0631(0.0097)	0-1
C	8	0.0626(0.0121)	0.0626(0.0131)	0

The animals with DCS due to the rapid decompression showed a significant decrease in PaO$_2$ ($P<0.05$) and increase in PaCO$_2$ ($P<0.05$, Table2). A significant relationship was found between the grade of Doppler signals and PaO$_2$ ($r=0.821$, $P<0.01$) or PaCO$_2$ ($r=0.856$, $P<0.01$). Although at 10 min postdive there was no statistical change in pH, O$_2$SAT and K$^+$ of serum, there was tendency to worsening in the animals that died earlier that 45 min postdive. Hemoconcentration did not appear during initial stage of acute DCS on the basis of no obvious change in the concentration of Hb (Table 2).

The autopsy contributed to evidence for diagnosis of DCS and VGE as well as to the determination of relationships among DCS, VGE and LDC. Gas bubbles in vessels could be observed only in most of the animals with acute DCS. We found a large drop of LDCco (average 63.64%) in the rabbits (N=10) suffering from severe DCS with VGE in large amounts and a small drop of LDCco (average 21.98%) in the animals (N=8) suffering from mild DCS with VGE in small amounts.

Table 2. Results of blood gas analysis in the animals with DCS

	Base line	Postdive
PaO2 (Kpa)	11.64 (0.26)	8.17 (2.21)*
PaCO2 (Kpa)	5.83 (0.69)	7.02 (0.90)*
O2SAT (%)	92.40 (1.40)	75.12 (16.94)
O2CT (Vol%)	14.92 (0.90)	12.23 (2.71)*
pH	7.39 (0.03)	7.28 (0.97)
K$^+$(MM/L)	3.88 (0.32)	5.23 (1.85)
Hb (g%)	11.42 (0.81)	11.57 (0.53)

Histological examination of the lungs of controls was unremarkable. Light microscopical examination showed mild degree congestion of the alveolar capillaries in animals of Group B. The prominent abnormalities were included in Group A. The degree of edema was mild to moderate and limited to the peribronchial region and adventitia of the pulmonary arteries. Histologically, almost all air emboli were restricted to the pulmonary arterial vessels (1500 to 100um in diam), several pulmonary arteries contained a single large air bubble (0.05 to 0.03 mm in diam) occupying the majority of the vascular lumen. Platelets and neutrophils accumulated around the air bubbles and formed intravascular clumps. The neutrophils also formed aggregates in the pulmonary arterial microvessels without air bubbles. The frozen tissue blocks showed fat emboli in the pulmonary arterioles in almost all cases of animals of Group A. With special stain a few white microthrombi locating the pulmonary arterioles and microvessels were observed. Occasionally, bone marrow emboli with megakaryocytes, histiocytes and myeloid cells were found squeezing into pulmonary arteries in some sections and arterioles in other sections. The alveolar epithelium appeared intact. Neither edema fluid nor extravasated cells exhibited in the alveolar spaces. Only one of the animals of Group A showed regional alveolar edema with slight degree.

DISCUSSION

Disordered gas exchange is an inevitable consequence of acute DCS in humans or animals. The mechanism or mechanisms responsible for this, however, have not been clearly delineated. Proposed mechanisms of hypoxemia have included right to left shunting, hyperventilation, inequality of ventilation and perfusion (V_A/Q), alveolar dead-space increase, broncho and/or pneumoconstriction, pulmonary hypertension and opening of a patent foramen ovale, pulmonary edema and low cardiac output. Although the contribution of these different mechanisms to the development of hypoxemia cannot be distinguished in this study, the basic mechanisms produced by bubble embolism to lung are reduction of perfusion in the embolized lung and increase of perfusion in non embolism lung, eventually cause impairment of diffusion. In this study, the animals suffering from acute DCS with hypoxemia showed a statistically significant decrease in LDCco and the decrease in LDCco significantly correlated to the grade of Doppler bubble signals, which indicate that the pulmonary gas diffusion was impaired by VGE. Histologically, it was very difficult to impute the impairment to increase in resistance of the alveolus-capillary to gas diffusion because of the lack any evidence of alveolar edema, whereas it was supported by the evidence of extensive pulmonary microembolism to impute the impairment to the reduction in the effective area for gas diffusion. Therefore it might be reasonable to consider that the decrease in LDC due to the reduction in the effective area for gas diffusion plays an important role in the pathogenesis of hypoxia in acute DCS.

Treatment of decompression sickness hawaiian style

Frank P. Farm, Jr., Edwin Hayashi and Edward L. Beckman, M.D.

A retrospective survey by personal interview of 44 of Hawaii's diving fishermen was carried out by the authors in 1981-82. Many of this group (22/44 = 50%) reported that they had used immediate in water recompression (IIWR) as a method of treatment for decompression sickness which it occurred while diving in the open ocean several hours away from the nearest decompression chamber.

These 22 divers who had used IIWR were subsequently re-interviewed in order to learn more about the technique used and the effectiveness of the procedure in ameliorating or curing decompression sickness (DCS). The data from this survey has been analyzed and the effectiveness of the IIWR treatment for decompression sickness has been evaluated.

The need for immediate recompression in the treatment of DCS has been emphasized for many years (U.S. Navy, 1963). However, when the U.S.N. recompression chambers at Pearl Harbor were made available for DCS treatment of Hawaii's diving fishermen (HDF) the emphasis for immediate recompression was skewed to immediate recompression in the recompression chamber. Hawaii's diving fishermen were thereafter admonished to come immediately to the recompression chamber at Pearl Harbor for treatment. However, the HDF netted and speared fish from small boats which they operated miles and hours away from the treatment chamber. They had learned that delay in treatment was detrimental to their recovery. They had learned, by trial and error, to treat DCS by immediate in water recompression (IIWR) using scuba. The effectiveness of this procedure was evaluated in this survey, and the parameters of IIWR treatments and their effectiveness were determined.

In order to understand the development of IIWR as a treatment for DCS, it is necessary to first understand the development of scuba diving in Hawaii.

The Cousteau-Gagnan self-contained underwater breathing apparatus was offered for sale in Honolulu in 1949. Skin divers who fished for monetary reward immediately recognized the commercial value of this device, which consisted of a gas bottle regulator and straps.

The waters around the Hawaiian Islands were clear and abounded with fish. Spearing or netting fish or collecting semi-precious coral by using scuba became a lucrative occupation. Upwards of 300 islanders used scuba diving either as a principal source of income or to augment other income. Of this group, more than 100 were still actively diving at the time of the survey of whom 44 were interviewed.

The ages of these divers varied from 61 to 31 years with a mean age of 42.5 years. The diving techniques developed by these divers are unique. They used small boats and carried many air tanks for diving and usually extra tanks for use in the case that one of the divers developed DCS. The survey revealed that the maximum number of dives made by any diver in one day was 12, with a mean value of 5.5 dives per day for all divers interviewed.

This explains why most experienced diver had amassed a total of over 23,400 dives up to the time of the survey. The mean number of dives made to the date of the survey was 11,000 per diver. The deepest air dive reported was 350 FSW on scuba. The mean maximum dive depth was 228 FSW. One group of black coral divers had worked a coral forest at over 300 FSW for over a month with 4-5 dives per week.

These HDF had learned by experience to make their deepest dive the first dive of the day, followed by less deep dives and then finished the day by making a so-called "scrape" dive to catch lobsters, octopus or reef fish at dive depths of 60 ft. or less.

Since this is a retrospective survey of personal experiences, it is apparent that unless the divers maintained a log which chronicled all of the incidents of DCS which they had experienced over the preceding 15-20 years, then these data would not necessarily be reliable. The divers did of course remember some specific incidents of DCS which they narrated. A few did keep logs, and these data were therefore available. It should also be remembered that the survey was of members of a small group of people, and they worked as teams. Therefore, each team member became a check against the others in augmenting, verifying or denying the memory of another. A further limitation in evaluation of IIWR results ensues from the lack of medicinal evaluation in most cases combined with the divers well known tendency for denial.

In addition, the records of treatment of DCS at the Pearl Harbor Treatment Centre were also available. Therefore by using these checks and balances we believe that the inferences derived from these data are essentially valid.

The divers interviewed reported the use of IIWR in the treatment of over 500 diving incidents of premonitory signs or frank decompression sickness. The treatment was successful except in 65 incidents. In 51 of these, divers reported significant improvement of bone pain but only to the point that they chose to "wait it out" or "bite the bullet" and used beer or aspirin as home remedies for 1-3 days until the ache subsided.

In addition there were 14 incidents of the total in which IIWR provided such inadequate recovery that further treatment was sought at the USN Recompression Treatment Chamber at Pearl Harbor. Of these, three (3) patients sought further relief from bone pain, ten (10) for spinal cord disease and one (1) for vestibular incoordination. Of these, nine (9) still had significant residuals following discharge after treatment by USN procedures. The magnitude of these residuals varied from persisting complete paraplegia to continuing vestibular incoordination.

The signs and symptoms which were relieved varied from the mild "Bends Type" DCS (primarily paid and aches around the shoulders and arms) to the more serious CNS conditions that included loss of vision, vestibular dizziness, loss of sensation, paraplegia, quadriplegia and clouding of consciousness. However, it should be noted that this type of DCS treatment apparently does not protect divers against the chronic form of decompression sickness of the bone, i.e. dysbaric osteonecrosis, a disease which many HDF have developed (Wade et al., 1978).

The water depths that were used for IIWR ranged from the deepest estimated depth of 85 FSW to the shallowest estimated depth of 25 FSW, with an average treatment depth of 41.3 FSW. IIWR times showed a high of 200 minutes and a low of 20 minutes, with an average decompression time of 63.7 minutes. Recompression depths of 30 FSW or less or for durations of 30 minutes or less usually did not prove effective in treating DCS.

CASE HISTORIES

One of the authors, (FF) has personally treated others several times and, likewise, has been treated himself by IIWR on two occasions. His personal treatments were for pain in the shoulder and arms. On one occasion after the onset of symptoms, he was rapidly taken to shallower water and two, one tank, "scrape" dives were made spearing fish in 55 to 45 FSW. Most of the pain disappeared immediately upon reaching depth, and relief continued while diving. He was very comfortable after the treatment dives.

In another incident (Figure 1), he initiated the IIWR of another diver who had made three dives ranging from 120 to 160 FSW. A few minutes after the third dive, the diver developed uncontrollable movements in both legs. The boat was already underway so FF piloted it toward shallower water. Within this few minutes the diver's lower body became paralyzed and he had no feeling from the nipple line down. He could not stand or move his lower extremities. A full tank of air was strapped to the victim who was still able to hold and breathe through the mouthpiece of the regulator. He was then lifted over the side of the boat and rolled into the water. FF was waiting in the water.

After checking the victim's breathing, he commenced pulling the disabled diver toward the bottom. No immediate benefit occurred at 40 FSW so FF towed the victim toward deeper water. In approximately 70 FSW, the victim started tugging and made noises and gave an "OK" hand signal. He further demonstrated that he had regained movement of his lower body.

The victim was instructed with hand signals to remain at the bottom holding onto or swimming around a large boulder. The boat was anchored directly above and a safety diver hung from a rope attached to the boat and watched from the surface while the victim recompressed. When the recompressing diver indicated low air pressure in his tank by engaging his reserve valve, the observing diver went to the bottom and exchanged tanks, thereby letting the victim have another full tank. The victim later ascended to 40 FSW and then to 20 FSW, where he stayed until the air supply was almost gone, and then surfaced. He felt a little tired that evening, but was observed to be walking normally and had had good return of strength in his legs and arms, as well as normal sensations throughout his body.

Another incident, which was reported by one of the divers interviewed, may explain why IIWR for the treatment of decompression sickness has been adopted by so many HDF. This incident was subsequently verified by other divers involved and by the County Coroner's Office. On this day of fishing, four divers were working in pairs at a site in about 165 to 180 FSW. Each pair alternated diving and made two dives each. Upon surfacing from the second dive, both divers on the second pair rapidly developed signs and symptoms of severe CNS decompression sickness. The driver of the boat and other diver headed for the dock some 30 minutes away. However, one diver refused to go and elected to undergo IIWR. He took two full scuba tank and told the boat driver to come back and pick him up after they got the other diver to the chamber. He was then rolled over the side of the boat.

The boat crew returned after two hours to pick him up, they found him swimming on the surface. He was asymptomatic and apparently cured of the disease. The other diver died of severe decompression sickness in the Med-Evac helicopter on the way to the recompression chamber.

SUMMARY

It should be emphasized that this survey reports on a treatment for decompression sickness which has been empirically developed over many years of use by a specific population at risk. This population is small, and the procedure is directed toward the treatment of a disease process which results from use of diving techniques used by HDF. These HDF employ many repetitive scuba dives with relatively short surface intervals. This IIWR technique for treatment of DCS has found to be effective in treatment of DCS as it afflicts HDF. It is proposed neither for universal use nor as a complete treatment.

In recent years we have encouraged HDF to use oxygen in addition to air in carrying out IIWR. We recommend that they carry a tank of oxygen (of 120 cu ft or more capacity) in their boat for use in treating decompression sickness in water. They have been instructed in the use of the Australian emergency underwater oxygen treatment (Edmonds et al., 1976) and the Hawaiian emergency in-water, air-oxygen recompression treatment (Beckman, 1981: Figure 2). They have been encouraged to carry the necessary equipment (tank of oxygen and regulator with 30 ft tether) with them on their boat and to initiate treatment by either method immediately if any crew member develops signs or symptoms which could be related to decompression sickness. They have been further advised to seek medical consultation at the Hyperbaric Treatment Centre immediately after receiving this treatment. The results from use of the air/oxygen recompression treatment table have been excellent for those who have used it. Unfortunately, the problems of procuring oxygen for use on small boats still limits its usefulness for HDF.

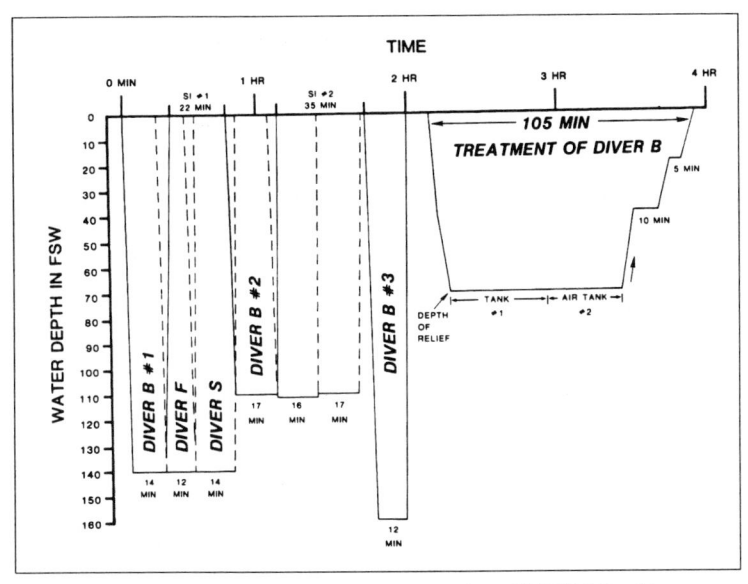

Figure 1 HDF repetitive dives which resulted in CNS/DCS with successful treatment by immediate in-water recompression

IMMEDIATE IN-WATER RECOMPRESSION

Conclusion:
IIWR using compressed air scuba has been found to be effective among H.D.F. in the treatment of all forms of DCS in its beginning stages.

Recommendations:
1. IIWR using the Hawaiian air/oxygen table is recommended for use by HDF in the treatment of DCS in its prodromal or earliest stages.
2. IIWR using compressed air scuba is acceptable for emergency use by HDF in treatment of DCS in its prodromal or earliest stages.
3. IIWR may be useful for emergency treatment of other divers who develop DCS when a recompression chamber is not immediately available.

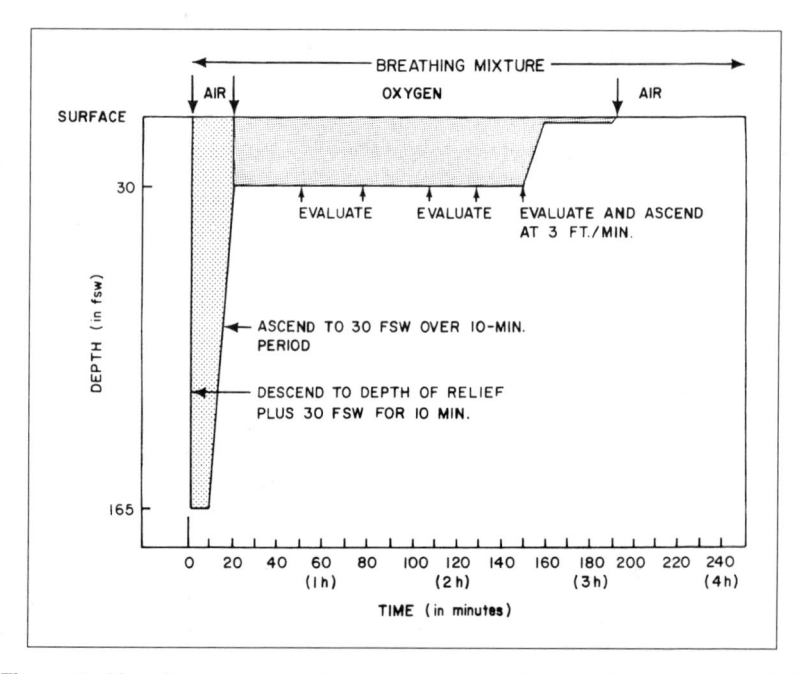

Figure 2. Hawaiian emergency in-water recompression schedule for treatment of DCS

REFERENCES

1. U.S. Navy Department, Section 3, 1963. U.S. Navy Diving Manual (NAVSHIPS 250-538). Best Publishing Company, Flagstaff, Arizona 86003-0100.
2. Wade, C.E., E.M. Hayashi, T.M. Cashman and E.L. Beckman. 1978. Incidence of dysbaric osteonecrosis in Hawaii's diving fishermen. Undersea Biomedical Research 5:2
3. Edmonds, C., C.F. Lowry and J. Pennefather. 1976. Diving and Subaquatic Medicine. 1st ed. New South Wales, Australia: Diving Medical Centre Publication.
4. Beckman, E.L. 1981. An emergency method for immediate in-water treatment of decompression sickness. Present at Alii Holo Kai Dive Club, June 30, 1981.

Changes of volume, K+, Na+, Cl-, and 17-OHCS of human urine during the simulated short-term air diving in dry chamber

G. T. Ni and H. J. Chen

Department of Naval Medicine, Second Military Medical University, Shanghai, China

Homeostatic responses to altered environment are complex and the physiology of stress has, to a large extent, been elucidated. However, is there a compression-decompression stress during an "adequate air dive?" And what is the effect of this stress on salt and water metabolism? We know very little and that is the purpose of our investigation.

MATERIALS AND METHOD

Subjects - Seven teachers and graduate students of Naval Diving Medicine (male, healthy, 22-42 years old) were selected for the experiment. One week before the experiment, all of them had a compression training at the pressure of 404 kpa and 606 kpa in order.

DIVE PROFILE

After a fast of 12 h and an arrest of drinking for 10 h, the divers were subjected to various conditions: condition A (at 202 kpa), condition B (at 404 kpa, 60 min, then decompressed to the surface within 60 min) and condition C (at 606 kpa, 60 min, then decompressed to the surface within 150 min). The temperature of the chamber was equal to that of environment and was maintained within +5°C during the compression-decompression treatment. The dive was conducted with subjects comfortably relaxed and awakened.

URINE COLLECTION AND CHEMICAL ANALYSIS

Urine was freely voided at the end of each time period (30 min), which was collected and used for analysis of 17-OHCS by Porter-Silber method, for the determination of K+, Na+ by flame spectrophotometry and for the measurement of Cl- by mercuric nitrate titration. Only values obtained at the 3rd time period were used as pre-compression controls.

RESULTS

Ions, volume and 17-OHCS variables are summarized in Table 1.

K^+. Beginning with the compression phase (period 4) of the dive there was a significant and sustained increase in K^+ concentration during sustained period of condition B (P<0.05) and condition C (P<0.01). At the same time, however, we also observed a secondary decrease in the ion concentrations during the decompression phase of condition C (P<0.05). No obvious change was obtained in condition A.

Na^+ and Cl^-. Our results showed a strange phenomenon, i.e. sea level treatment resulted in an elevation of those two kinds of ion concentrations (Na^+, P<0.05; Cl^-, P<0.01) during the decompression periods.

Volume of urine. There was a tendency of increase and a subsequent restoration in urine flow during compression and decompression periods respectively. But this alteration was not statistic significant.

17 OHCS. Urine contents of 17-OHCS were not affected by the compression-decompression treatment.

DISCUSSION

From the present study we suggest that significant stress response do not seem to be involved in "adequate air dive," since urine contents of 17-OHCS were not affected by the "compression-decompression stress." And the changes of K^+, Na^+ and Cl^- might be attributed to the mechanism other than the stress. The precise mechanism is worth further investigation.

Table 1. Response of ions, volume and 17 OHCS

	Pressure (kpa)	3	4	5	6	7	8	9	10
Volume of urine (Y%)	101	100	101.5±5.5	109.0±10.5	105.0±13.1	95.4±10.2	90.6±11.6	87.4±12.6	
	404	100	118.3±36.3	153.6±93.8	140.6±92.0	95.9±25.1			
	606	100	118.0±24.2	148.6±94.2	101.9±40.0	104.2±77.9	98.1±68.7	77.6±21.4	80.1±24.4
K^+ (Y%)	101	100	101.0±11.3	104.3±16.5	101.7±23.1	99.8±24.7	100.1±24.5	96.5±24.9	
	404	100	122.7±23.1	134.8±34.6*	127.5±24.9	101.7±20.0			
	606	100	129.9±25.6*	144.9±31.1**	107.5±22.6	81.9±22.7	77.5±24.7*	73.2±19.8*	75.5±19.7*
Na^+ (Y%)	101	100	103.9±5.1	113.7±9.7*	109.0±12.5	100.4±9.4	96.3±12.6	96.3±12.6	96.7±16.3
	404	100	104.5±16.6	90.8±25.6	90.0±25.6	93.5±23.8			
	606	100	108.8±21.3	82.1±22.0	74.4±16.8*	82.1±22.5*	86.9±29.3	84.9±24.0	91.9±35.1
Cl^- (Y%)	101	100	102.8±3.9	111.0±6.7**	106.6±10.5	97.7±10.4	92.1±10.4	89.8±14.6	
	404	100	107.4±14.8	93.6±14.8	93.6±21.7	91.7±25.7	95.0±26.4		
	606	100	107.2±15.9	80.8±14.1	68.0±14.9**	72.0±20.6*	75.2±23.1	76.1±20.9*	81.8±25.0
17-OHCS (Y%)	101	100	113.2±27.3	113.2±27.3	105.6±20.7	105.6±20.7			
	404	100	102.4±30.9	102.4±30.9	90.1±20.7	90.1±20.7			
	606	100	90.0±43.4	90.0±43.4	98.3±103.1	98.3±103.1			

(n=7. **: P<0.01, *: P<0.05), (Y% = values/controls • 100%)

An investigation for evaluation of different recompression treatment tables of air decompression sickness by means of agarose gel bubble technique

Hang, Rong-Chung Lian and Qin-Lin

Second Military Medical College, Shanghai, China.

There is a lot of re-compression treatment tables for air decompression sickness. Which table amongst them is the best? We infer that agarose gel bubble technique may be used to evaluation of different recompression treatment tables for air decompression sickness rapidly and objectively. Thus we conducted this investigation for evaluating recompression treatment tables of Russia, U.S. Navy, Naval Medical Research Institute of China PLA and our Department.

MATERIALS AND METHODS

1. Preparation of agarose gel

The agarose powder used preparation of agarose gel was one of the reagent grade made in China and the buffer was tris (Hydroxymethyl) aminome thane. In order to form adequate amount of bubbles, we selected a prescription in which the concentration of the agarose sol was 0.8%, and the pH of tris solution was adjusted to 9.0. However the pH of the agarose solution was 8.1. The agarose sol was then poured into a lot of counting cells made of transparent plastics. Each counting cell was 0.25 cm. The average bubble numbers in the agarose gel of one counting cell formed normal decompression after simulated diving was 5.5±4.

2. Preparation of the agarose gel bubble models of simulated decompression sickness and their controls.

First, we selected 10 cases of decompression sickness. Among them 6 were type I, and 4 type II. These cases have been separately treated by the recompression treatment table of our department, Naval Medical research Institute of China PLA, U.S. Navy, or of Russia. We prepared separately agarose gel models of decompression sickness as experimental groups. The agarose gel models of each case of decompression sickness were divided into A,B,C, and D experimental groups, so as to treated separately by the cells in one experimental group. Conducting simulated diving in a chamber with the diving depth and bottom time of a certain diving related to the onset of corresponding case of decompression sickness, but decompression according to an adequate schedule of U.S. standard decompression table. We made its control group which consisted of eighteen counting cells.

The temperatures in the chamber were maintained at 25±3°C during the course of the compression-decompression.

The bubbles formed in agarose gel of every counting cell of experimental groups and control groups were observed and calculated with the aid of stereomicroscope. Because the forms of bubbles looked like spindles, we measured their long diameters and short diameters of some bubbles localized a certain area by a vernier caliper.

3. "Recompression treatment" of experimental groups and observation of "curative effect"

The A.B.C. and C experimental groups of each case were separately treated in the chamber by a certain therapeutic schedule of a recompression treatment table amongst the four recompression treatment tables mentioned above. The therapeutic schedule was selected in light of respective related rules of the four recompression treatment tables. The variation of the number of the bubbles in agarose gel of every counting cell of experimental groups were observed during the recompression courses. After decompression, observed again, and compared with each other.

RESULTS AND DISCUSSION

1. The averages of bubbles in the agarose gel of every counting cells of the experimental groups before the recompression treatment were greater than those after the recompression treatment and those in the related control groups, but the averages of bubbles in the experimental groups were all less than those before the recompression treatment and 35 of 40 experimental groups were less than those in related control groups (Table 1: P.0.01).

This result indicated that the agarose gel as simulated tissue may reflect the characteristics of actual tissues in some degree. In the same condition averages of bubbles formed in the agarose gel increase with the rapid decompression. The recompression treatment can make the bubbles decrease. It follows Boyle-Mariotte's law and Henry's law. If it is certain that the averages of bubbles are in the related control groups do not cause decompression sickness, the used therapeutic schedules of the four recompression treatment tables are satisfying according to the curative effects. The results are consistent with those using the therapeutic schedules to treat the cases.

2. It was different that treating the four experiment groups of the same case separately by different recompression treatment table mentioned above caused variation of respective average. The curative effect of recompression treating with the therapeutic schedules of the recompression treatment table of Naval Medical Research Institute of China PLA was the best amongst the four treatment tables. The averages of bubbles in the experimental groups after treating with this recompression treatment table were all less than those

in the related control groups, and the decompression time of every therapeutic schedule is not the longest. On the contrary, the averages of bubbles treating with the recompression treatment table of Russia were not all less that those in the related control groups and one of them was still greater than that in the related control group. This arouses our suspicion that to vary stop time at certain stop stations in recompression treatment table of Russia is necessary.

3. The average of bubbles in 3 of 4 experimental group of case No 9 were still greater than those of the related control group after recompression treatment.

It may be attributed to the diving depth. The diving depth related the onset of case No 9 is the deepest amongst those of the 10 cases. Right away the case No 9 was a type II of DCS and the curative effect of recompression treatment was "on the mend". This reminds us to select recompression schedule conscientiously to DCS caused by the deeper diving.

4. The bubbles in the agarose gel of experimental groups disappeared all or in part and the sizes of the remaining bubbles were constricted under the therapeutic pressure, but the sizes of the remaining bubbles after recompression treatments approached those before recompression treatment.

The rules of movement of the inert gas in the body were experimentally investigated with agarose gel as a simulated tissue. It can get objective conclusion from two important sides those are diffusion and solvation of the gas in the tissues. Of course, perfusion of the blood has certain influence, but it usually accelerates bubble to disappear. Therefore that this investigation did not involve the perfusion may not hinder safety in evaluation of the recompression treatment tables.

Table 1. The comparison of averages of bubbles between experimental groups and control groups.

cases No.	simulated contral groups	A pre-recomp.	A post-recomp.	B pre-recomp.	B post recomp.	C pre recomp.	C post recomp.	D pre recomp.	D post recomp.
1	1.3±1.4	25.5±3.7	3.0±1.9	26.6±4.2	0.16±0.3	24.4±2.7	0.5±0.9	23.1±3.5	0.2±0.7
2	4.1±2.4	27.7±5.9	3.6±2.7	28.3±4.6	2.7±1.9	28.5±3.8	0.2±0.4	26.0±4.0	0
3	6.3±2.6	30.4±4.3	6.3±6.5	22.3±2.8	0	21.2±3.1	0.2±0.9	39.3±6.0	0.1±0.4
4	17.3±5.6	99.4±8.6	0	150.9±7.0	0	110.9±8.1	0	115.3±9.3	0
5	17.3±3.1	38.4±6.1	21±4.7	41.7±6.9	0.16±0.38	44.7±6.7	5.3±2.6	41.5±3.5	7.2±0.3
6	14.5±4.1	81±37.6	0.05±0.23	64.3±19.9	2±4.7	86.1±37.6	0	99.7±0.9	0.05±0.23
7	78.2±3.2	48.3±12	0.1±0.3	30.5±8.6	1±3.2	28.5±18	1.8±2.3	52±7.1	0
8	9.5±2.9	56.7±7.5	0.2±0.5	101.5±10.5	0.1±0.4	28.5±5.3	0	21.9±8.6	0
9	8.4±5.9	71.7±17.6	25.4±6.5	43.2±8.2	7.7±3.2	34.8±17.4	18.1±5.5	37±6.6	21.3±2.9
10	6.5±1.9	60.1±16.5	1±2.6	65.4±20.5	0.2±0.4	51.5±17.1	2.8±2.3	44±6.4	2.6±2.9

REFERENCES

1. Mano Y, et al: Undersea Biomed Res 9 (1) : 45, 1982.
2. Strauss RH, et al: Isobaric Bubble Growth: A consequence of Altering Atmospheric Gas Science 186, PP 443-444 1974.
3. Yono K, et al: The Bulletin of Tokyo Medical and Dental University 26, PP 197-212, 1979.
4. Miyamoto T, et al: The Bulletin of Tokyo Medical and Dental University 27, PP 96-109, 1980.
5. Mano Y et al, Under water physiology VIII, 181-200, 1986.
6. Ni, GT. (Editor), Practical Diving Medicine, PP 99-110, People's Health Press, 1980. (In Chinese).
7. Gong, JH. (Editor) Diving Medicine, Edition Princeps, PP 186-258, People's Military Medical Press 1985. (In Chinese).
8. Hang, RC. Application of Agarose Gel Bubble technic on Investigation for Preventing DCS, Military Medical Branch Abroad Medicine, 6, PP 343-345, 1985 (Chinese).
9. Li, YC. Experimental Investigation of Simulated Human Tissues by Agarose Gel Models, Ocean Underwater Engineering (4), 28-31, 1985. (In Chinese).
10. Hang, RC. et al. 7810 Recompression Treatment Table for Air Diving DCS and Its Effect on Preliminary Probation, Rescue and Diving 1, 36-43 1986. (In Chinese)

Hyperbaric oxygen in the management of skeletal muscle-compartment syndrome

Michael B. Strauss, M.D., F.A.C.S., A.A.O.S.[*], Diana A. Greenburg, R.N., M.S.N.[**] and George B. Hart, M.D., F.A.C.S.[***]

[*]Associate director, [**]Manager, [***]Baromedical department,
Memorial Medical Center, 2801 Atlantic Avenue,
Long Beach, CA 90801-1428

INTRODUCTION

Even though we have improved awareness and ability to diagnosis the skeletal muscle-compartment syndrome (SMCS), problems still exist in its management. For example, a single interstitial fluid compartment pressure measurement does not tell whether the SMCS is in its lag phase, is plateauing, is worsening, or is resolving. Second, as the compartment volume enlarges from swelling, compartment pressures initially increase slowly. Once the compartment is maximally distended pressures rise rapidly with further swelling due to decreased compliance. [1] The clinician may be led into a false sense of security if his/her treatment is based on the rate of the initial changes in pressure. Third, there are no intermediate interventions between observation and surgical decompression. Fourth, once a major neuropathy develops, the chances for recovery are less than 15%. [2] Finally, animal studies show that hypotension very significantly lowers the threshold pressure for the compartment syndrome. [3]

Based on our knowledge of the pathophysiology of the SMCS and the appreciation of these problems, we proposed that hyperbaric oxygen (HBO) would be a useful intervention. To test our hypothesis we collaborated with the Department of Orthopedic Surgery, University of California, San Diego on compartment syndrome studies using a dog model. The studies conclusively demonstrated that HBO ameliorated the compartment syndrome in this model. [4,5,6] To date no clinical studies have been published on the effects of HBO on the SMCS. The paper summarizes our experiences using HBO as an adjunct to manage this problem.

MATERIALS AND METHODS

A retrospective analysis was done of all patients referred to the Baromedical Department at Memorial Medical Center, Long Beach, California with a diagnosis of SMCS between 1979 and 1986. Eighteen patients received hyperbaric oxygen treatments. Their ages ranged from 6 to 69 with a mean of

32. Eighty-five percent were male and 15% female. There were three general causes of the SMCS: injury, post vein harvesting for coronary bypass surgery and intercurrent illness (Table 1). Swelling was the presenting sign in all patients. Pain was a significant feature in eight-five percent, and present in all but the obtunded patients. Pain aggravated by passive stretch and neuropathy were present in 61% and 50% of the patients respectively. Ten patients (55%) were given HBO without surgical decompression of the compartment. Eight patients received HBO postoperatively either because of anticipated wound healing problems, further loss of tissues, neuropathy, or combinations of these. The majority of HBO treatments were for 90 minute durations two to three time a day at pressures of two atmospheres absolute.

RESULTS

In the ten patients, who did not undergo surgical decompression, the SMCS resolved with HBO treatments. Five patients in this group had compartment pressure measurements. In three of the five (60%), the pressures were high enough that surgical decompression would have been recommended if there had not been other mitigating circumstances. These circumstances included intercurrent myocardial infarction, immediate nonavailability of the operating room, and threatened tissue slough from infiltration of medicines. In two other patients the compartment pressures were 20mmHg or less but HBO was started because of tense swelling, pain, pain with passive stretch, and neuropathy. One patient with polytrauma expired from causes other than the compartment syndrome.

In the eight patients that received hyperbaric oxygen treatments after surgical decompression, all according to the attending surgeon's comments, were benefited. Benefits included edema reduction, survival of marginal tissues, and preservation of compromised flaps at the time of closure. These accelerated recovery and reduced hospital stays. Four patients in this group had neuropathies including two with foot drop. In all four the neuropathies resolved. Two additional patients had tissue losses. One from a gun shot would and one from debridement of nonviable muscles.

The number of hyperbaric oxygen treatments varied markedly between those patients who received HBO without surgical decompression and those who received HBO treatments postoperatively (Table 2). The mean number of HBO treatments for the HBO patients who did not have surgical decompression was 12 as compared to 36 for the patients who started HBO after surgery. The number of HBO treatments was also influenced by the cause of the SMCS. The greatest number of HBO treatments occurred in those patients where the SMCS developed secondary to an underlying disease (e.g. gas gangrene, deep vein thrombosis). The fewest number of HBO treatments were given to those patients who compartment syndrome were of an ischemic rather than traumatic origin as after vein harvesting for coronary artery bypass surgery. In the post trauma group the number of HBO treatments varied with the degree of injury. The most HBO treatments were given to the patients with combined crush injuries and fractures. The HBO treatments were well tolerated in all but two (11%) patients. For one patient HBO was stopped because of claustrophia after two treatments while for the second patient it was stopped during the first treatment because of an anxiety reaction possible seizure. This latter patient's compartment pressure measured only mmHg but a neuropathy was present. Neither had subsequent surgical decompression.

DISCUSSION AND CONCLUSIONS

The findings in this retrospective study are consistent with the known mechanisms of hyperbaric oxygen and the published laboratory studies. The maximum benefit of HBO appeared to be in those cases where surgical decompression had not been done. Where it had been done HBO was utilized as adjunct to management of the complications resulting from the compartment syndrome. Those patients who started HBO after surgical intervention had on the average three times the number of HBO treatments as the patients who had HBO without surgical decompression.

The full role of HBO is the SMCS is yet to be established. It is not a substitute for surgical decompression in cases where compartment pressures are markedly elevated, neuropathy is present, or both. The sooner HBO treatments are started the more likely it will be beneficial. The mechanisms of HBO interrupt the ischemia edema, cycle which causes progression of the SMCS. In no case did HBO worsen the compartment syndrome symptoms or compromise the other care given to the patient.

Table 1. Compartment syndrome: Etiology

	INJURY	SURGERY*	ILLNESS
Number	13	3	2
Percent	72	17	11
Age Range	16-44	53-69	6-9
Mean Range	29	61	7.5

*Post vein harvesting for coronary artery bypass

Table 2. Compartment syndrome

NUMBER OF HBO RXS	
NO SURGERY (10 PATIENTS)	POST-OP (8 PATIENTS)
RESOLVED (7 PATIENTS) Range: 4 to 18 Mean: 12 STOPPED PREMATURELY* (2 Patients) Range: 1 to 2 Mean: 1.5 EXPIRED (1 Patient) 9	Range: 7 to 63 Mean: 36

* (1) Claustrophobia
  (2) Possible seizure, anxiety reaction

REFERENCES

1. Hargens AR, Akeson WH, Mubarak SJ, et al: Fluid balance within the canine anterolateral compartment and its relationship to compartment syndromes. J Bone Jt Surg 60-A:499-505, 1978.
2. Bradley EL III: The anterior tibial compartment syndrome. Surg Gynecol Obstet 136:289-297, 1973.
3. Zweifach SS, Hargens, AR, Evans, KL, et al: Skeletal muscle necrosis in pressurized compartments associated with hemorrhagic hypotension. J Trauma 20:941-947, 1980.
4. Strauss MB, Hargens, AR, Gershuni DH, et al: Delayed use of hyperbaric oxygen for treatment of a model anterior compartment syndrome. J Bone Jt Surg 65-A: 656-662, 1983.
5. Strauss MB, Hargens AR, Gershuni DH, et al: Delayed use of hyperbaric oxygen for treatment of a model anterior compartment syndrome. J Orthopedic Res 4:108-111, 1986.
6. Skyhar MJ, Hargens AR, Strauss MB, et al: Hyperbaric oxygen reduces edema and necrosis of skeletal muscle in compartment syndromes associated with hemorrhagic hypotension. J Bone Jr Surg 68-A; 1218-1224, 1986.

Hyperbaric oxygen therapy in the treatment of osteomyelitis

M. Kawashima, H. Tamura and K. Takao

Kawashima Orthopedic Hospital

Osteomyelitis is common, and despite modern advances in antibiotic therapy, may still cause disastrous disability. The problems and the disappointments associated with its treatment are well known to orthopedic surgeons. Closed irrigation suction is one of the best methods for treating osteomyelitis therapy, but if it fails to arrest the infection and prevent recurrence, the infection may eventually become chronic.

The lack of tissue vascularity and bone sclerosis prevent oxygen, antibiotics, and nutrients from reaching diseased areas in appropriate concentrations. Bingham and Hart demonstrated that hyperbaric oxygen, at a pressure of 2 or 3 atmospheres absolute (ATA), is bacteriostatic and in some instances bacteriocidal.

Hyperbaric oxygen increases osteoblast and osteoclast activity.

Vascular proliferation is stimulated by repeated exposure to hyperbaric oxygen for periods of ten days or more.

From 1982 to 1985, 70 patients with osteomylitis were treated by hyperbaric oxygenation (HBO).

The purpose of this paper is to report out experiences with these patients.

METHODS AND MATERIALS

HBO treatment was conducted at an equivalent of 2 atmospheres absolute (2 ATA or 29.4 psi), with patients breathing 100 per cent oxygen by face mask or closed loop hood assembly for one hour once daily for at least 4 weeks before and after the operation.

The steel multiplace hyperbaric chamber accommodates eight ambulatory patients. Pressure is computer controlled.

The effect of oxygenation was estimated from the transcutaneous oxygen pressure ($tcPO_2$).

Table 1 shows the $tcPO_2$ before HBO and during HBO. Average $tcPO_2$ before HBO at one ATA was 74mmHg and average $tcPO_2$ during HBO was 659mmHg.

From 1982 through 1985, 70 cases of osteomyelitis were treated of which 36 were treated by closed irrigation combined with HBO therapy, and 34 were treated by HBO therapy only, with a minimum follow-up of one year. Thirty eight patients had hematogenous infection, and 32 patients had traumatic or postoperative infection. Table 2 shows age distribution of the treated patients. Infection was localized at the sites noted in Table 3. A bacteriologic analysis was made on materials obtained from 70 cases (Table 4).

RESULTS

Excellent results with complete objective and subjective healing (Success) were noted in all 36 patients treated by irrigation suction combined with HBO therapy (Table 5).

Excellent results were noted in 23 of the 34 patients treated by HBO only (Table 6), improvement with either objective or subjective healing followed by later breakdown, or with decreased drainage and lessening of pain in 7, and recurrence in the remaining 4. The average number of treatment hours was 58.2, with a range from 4 to 240 (Table 7).

CASE REPORTS

Case 1: A 21 year old woman was admitted to hospital, with a chronic osteomyelitis of mandible. Two curratage operations and one bone grafting had been performed in other hospitals, but she complained continuous pain and swelling. HBO therapy was started, and in the following thirty days she received 26 treatments. During this period there was resolution of swelling, and she was relieved from pain. After 60 treatments, the sites healed completely.

Case 2: A 50 year old woman sustained an open fracture to the right tibia. She was originally treated with debridement and antibiotics in other hospitals. The patient developed a purulent discharge from the right tibia, with x-ray evidence of osteomyelitis. Three operations were performed, and discharge continued. The would healed after 30 HBO therapy. Bone graft with plate fixation and closed irrigation were performed for delayed bone union. Electric stimulation was performed for accelerating the bone union. Six months after, bone union was confirmed and wound healed completely.

Case 3: A 66 year old man was admitted, with a chronic osteomyelitis of right femur. The pain and the drainage from osteomyelitis had not responded to repeated debridements and antibiotic treatment for 43 years. Debridement was performed. We made a new irrigation system to prevent the obstruction of the drainage tube. Closed irrigation with this new circuit system was performed for 21 days after operation. Then 60 HBO therapy was performed. Finally, he became free of pain and drainage ceased.

Case 4: A 74 year old man had a long-standing history of chronic osteomyelitis of right femur. The pain and discharge had not responded to repeated debridements and antibiotic treatment for 20 years. After 60 HBO therapy, he became free of pain and drainage.

Case 5: A 52 year old man sustained open fracture of the left tibia. Discharge continued for 24 years. A skin defect was seen at the upper tibia. After debridement and muscle pedicular skin graft were performed, 30 HBO therapy was carried out. He became free of pain and discharge completely.

DISCUSSION

At the point when basic treatment of the infection fails, osteomyelitis may be considered refractory. Bingham and Hart noted that small sequestra can resorb under hyperbaric oxygen treatment, but persistent sequestra should be surgically removed. Direct prolonged lavage with solutions containing antibiotics was first reported by Smith Petersen in 1945.

Compere, in 1962, recommended the addition of Alevaire to the irrigation fluid. We reported a series of 232 patients treated with 256 closed irrigation suction procedures. Of these, 226 (88.3%) were treated successfully, 7 (2.7%) were improved and 23 (9.0%) were failures. Closed irrigation suction therapy is generally thought to be one of the best methods for treating osteomyelitis.

Hamblem (1968) reported that hyperbaric oxygen promoted the healing of rat tibia infected with Staphylococcus aureus. Goldhaver (1958) noted that exposing cultures of young mouse calvaria to hyperbaric oxygen bone caused resorption followed by osteoid tissue formation. Shaw and Basset (1967) demonstrated in tissue cultures that maximum osteogenesis and collagen-fiber formation occur under increased oxygen tension. Hunt (1965) demonstrated that HBO increases fibroblastic activity, probably by increasing the rate of synthesis of adenosine triphosphate in hyperoxic tissue. This results in the mitosis and migration of fibroblasts, with concomitant increases in the formation of collagen matrix necessary for capillary ingrowth. Mader (1978) demonstrated that HBO was as effective as cephalosporins in controlling experimentally induced staphylococcus osteomyelitis in rabbits. The investigators concluded that the value of HBO lies in its enhancing leucocyte functions rather than its ability to suppress microorganisms. These laboratory studies support the clinical results. Sippel (1969) reported treated a patient with osteomyelitis of the mandible with HBO therapy. Two years after the treatment, the patient had not exacerbation and wore complete dentures without difficulty.

Depenbusch (1972) reported excellent results with complete objective and subjective healing of refractory osteomyelitis in 35 of 50 patients. Bingham and Hart reported that of 70 patients with refractory osteomyelitis treated with HBO, all were improved and 63% remained free of disease.

Our experience also confirms that HBO is very effective in treating osteomyelitis. We are convinced that HBO is a valuable supplemental therapy, which combined with closed irrigation suction can produce superior results.

ACKNOWLEDGEMENT

It is a pleasure to thank Professor Tamikazu Amako for his valuable suggestions and encouragement.

Table 1. Trans cutaneous oxygen pressure of patients with osteomyelitis

Case No.	1 ATA	before HBO at 2 ATA	after HBO at 2 ATA
1	60mmHg	79mmHg	480mmHg
2	87mmHg	155mmHg	790mmHg
3	74mmHg	140mmHg	674mmHg
4	76mmHg	120mmHg	690mmHg
average	74mmHg	124mmHg	659mmHg

Table 2. Age Distribution of the treated Patients

Age	Male	Female	Total
0 - 9	0	0	0
10 - 19	3	1	4
20 - 29	4	5	9
30 - 39	11	1	12
40 - 49	8	0	8
50 - 59	10	7	17
60 - 69	9	5	14
70 -	5	1	6
Total	50	20	70

Table 3. Sites of Osteomyelitis

	Male	Female	Total
Mandible	3	6	9
Sternum	0	2	2
Radius	2	0	2
Fingers	1	0	1
Pelvis	2	0	2
Femur	14	5	19
Tibia	27	2	29
Foot	4	2	6
Total	53	17	70

Table 4. Microbiology

Microorganisms	Hematogenous	Traumatic	Total
Staphyl.aureus	8	6	14
Staphyl.epidermidis	1	2	3
Pseudomonas aeruginosa	4	6	10
Serratia, M.	0	1	1
Tuberclosis	4	0	4
Streptococcus	1	0	1
Bacteroides	0	1	1
Klebsiela	0	1	1
unclear	13	7	20
negative	6	9	15
Total	37	33	70

Table 5. Results of Irrigation - Suction associated with HBO Therapy

	Hematogenous Infection		Traumatic Infection		Total Infections	
Results	Number	%	Number	%	Number	%
Success	21	100	15	100	36	100
Improvement	0		0		0	
Failure	0		0		0	
Total	21		15		36	

Table 6. Results of HBO Therapy only

	Hematogenous Infection		Traumatic Infection		Total Infections	
Results	Number	%	Number	%	Number	%
Success	15	88.2	8	47.1	23	67.6
Improvement	1	5.9	6	35.3	7	20.6
Failure	1	5.9	3	17.6	4	11.8
Total	17		17		34	

Table 7. The Treatment Hours and Cases

Hours	Cases
0 - 19	10
20 - 39	24
40 - 59	10
60 - 79	10
80 - 99	4
more than 100 hours	12
Total	70

REFERENCES

1. Bingham EL, Hart GB. Hyperbaric oxygen treatment of refractory osteomyelitis. Postgrad. Med. 1977;61:70-76.
2. Smith Petersen MN. Local chemotherapy with primary closure of septic wounds by means of drainage and irrigation cannulae. J. Bone Joint Surg. 1945;27(4):562-571.
3. Mitra RN, Grace EJ. Further studies on the treatment of chronic osteomyelitis with topical detergent antibiotics therapy. Antbiot Ann. 1956-1957;4:455-466.
4. Compere EL, Treatment of osteomyelitis and infected wounds by closed irrigation with a detergent-antibiotic solution. Acta Orthop Scand. 1962;32:324-333.
5. Kawashima M, Tamura H. Topical therapy in orthopedic infection. Orthopedics. 1984;7:1592-1598.
6. Hamblem DL. Hyperbaric oxygenation. Its effect on experimental staphylococcal osteomyelitis in rats. J Bone Joint Surg. 1968;50-A:1129-1141.
7. Goldhaber P. The effect of hyperoxia on bone resorption in tissue culture. Arch Pathol Lab Med. 1958;66:635.
8. Shaw JL, Basset CA. The effect of varying oxygen concentrations on osteogenesis and embryonic cartilage in vitro. J Bone Joint Surg. 1967;49-A:73-80.
9. Hunt TK, Zerderfeldt B, Goldstick TK. Oxygen and healing. Am J Surg. 1969;49-A:73-80.
10. Mader JT, Guckian JC, Glass DL, Reinarz JA. Therapy with hyperbaric oxygen for experimental osteomyelitis due to staphylococcus aureus in rabbits. J. Infect Dis. 1978;138:312-318.
11. Sippel WH, Nyberg CD, Alvis HJ. Hyperbaric oxygen as an adjunct to the treatment of chronic osteomyelitis of the mandible. J Oral Surg., 1969;27:739-741.
12. Depenbusch FL, Thompson RE, Hart GB. Use of hyperbaric oxygen in the treatment of refractory osteomyelitis. A preliminary report. J Trauma. 1972;12:807-812.

Intracranial Abscesses

Rationales for a Therapeutic Approach by Hyperbaric Oxygenation

Lampl, L., Frey, G., Albert F.*, and Dietze T.

Department of Anaesthesiology and Intensive Care Medicine
(Head: OTA PD Dr. Bock)
*Department of Neurosurgery
(Head: OTA Prof. Dr. Oldenkott)
Federal Armed Forces Hospital,
D - 7900 Ulm/Donau,
Federal Republic of Germany

Intracranial abscesses account for the most serious infections of the human organism. Though these disorders are comparatively rare with approximately three to five admissions per year at large medical centers (4), the mortality ranges from 9.7% to 35.7% (2,4). A high percentage of surviving patients suffer from various neurologic deficits, mainly epileptic in origin.

Progresses in antibiotic therapy and especially the early and exact diagnosis by computed tomography has led to a significant reduction in mortality over the last few years. Over the same period of time, however, the number of patients suffering from intracranial abscesses as a complication of immunosuppression has increased. All in all, mortality remains to be considerably high.

Parallel to this development, knowledge of the bacteriological origin of intracranial abscesses grew more profound. Anaerobic germs among the bacteria isolated account for some 80% of the organisms responsible, depending on the culturing technique applied (2, 9, 11)! Anaerobic germs being predominant in intracranial abscesses is a fact commonly accepted throughout world literature today.

BROOK in the Journal of Neurosurgery (1) gives a very clear and detailed differentiation of the bacteriological findings in the 19 children with intracranial abscesses: in 63.2% exclusively anaerobic germs were found, whereas exclusively anaerobic organisms existed in only 10.5% of the specimens. In 26.3% there proved to be miscellaneous cultures, containing aerobic as well as anaerobic bacteria. The arrangements of brain abscesses on the one hand and subdural empyema on the other revealed no difference in regard to the predominance of the anaerobic organisms responsible (see Fig. 1).

All these bacteriologic results, cited by the international literature, including the Australian one (2), provide profound arguments for the application of HBO in such cases. On the opposite they illustrate the difficulties of effective antibiotic therapy, as well. The commonly known problems of antibiotic availability on the scene of infection are to be mentioned only briefly; they concern the permeability of the blood-brain-barrier on the one hand and the activity of the substances within the abscess itself on the other hand.

Dangers of different nature may result from the expansive growth of an intracranial abscess itself or from its perifocal edema. Thereby secondary lesions of brain tissue may result, or at worst, life threatening increases of intracranial pressure (ICP) may arise. The influence of hyperbaric oxygenation on increased ICP has been known for a long time (Jacobson and co-workers, Miller and Ledingham, qu. from 13). Summarized, hyperbaric oxygenation is able to reduce an increased ICP, especially in combination with hypocapnic hyperventilation. HBO directly acts on auto-regulated small blood vessels. The elevated arterial oxygen tension results in a vasoconstriction with a decrease of the cerebral blood flow, and consecutively in a reduction of an increased ICP. In addition to the common normobaric hypocapnic hyperventilation, HBO guarantees the sufficient oxygen delivery to potentially hypoxic brain areas. This is said to be of major importance in the prevention, respectively in the treatment of secondary brain damaging processes (3,7).

Two factors limit the benefit of HBO: rebound phenomena after ending the hyperoxygenation (13) and a reincrease of the cerebral blood-flow if a pressure of two bars is exceeded, as was depicted by OHTA 1984 at Long Beach (12).

According to common opinion, ours included, HBO in such critical cases must not be considered as a substitute for intensive care, but it should be seen as an enhancement, especially with non-responders to conventional therapy. We like to emphasize that HBO is only an integrated component of a comprehensive and continuous intensive care treatment. This is comparable to the four therapeutic pillars of the gas gangrene management, which are intensive care itself, the administration of antibiotics, surgery, and of course HBO (5). Depleting the structure of just one of these pillars might easily lead to the collapse of the entire therapeutic building.

Adapted to our patients with increased ICP due to intracranial suppurative processes, this mean hypocapnic hyperventilation, the continuous administration of drugs (such as adrenergic agents, barbiturates, antibiotics), the balanced fluid and electrolyte substitution, the head-up position and the invasive monitoring of vital functions. Depending on the chamber equipment used, there always will be need of plenty of improvisation.

Fig. 2 illustrates the development of the life threatening ICP in a 31 year old patient suffering from multiple abscesses throughout the entire left hemisphere (11), undergoing seven sessions of HBO according to the classic schedule of BOEREMA (qu. from 5). Remarkably, after the first session the endangering ICP-peaks had already disappeared, and after three days ICP remained constantly within normal limits. The patient finally was discharged from our hospital in good health with only slight neurologic disabilities.

We consider this to be a crucial indication, that hyperbaric oxygen in such cases does not provide only a symptomatic effect on increased ICP-levels, as described in different studies mentioned about (12, 13, 15). At this point the causative effect of HBO becomes obvious, by means of the simultaneous and essential destruction of the responsible, mostly anaerobic organisms generating the suppurative process and, secondary to this, the brain edema. In addition to the well-known and widely documented therapeutic effect of HBO on anaerobic as well as miscellaneous infections (5), we regard this a basic and crucial rationale for hyperbaric treatment of intracranial abscesses.

Further basic mechanisms of hyperbaric oxygen, for example the enhancement of leukocyte microbial killing (6) are well-known to the audience and therefore just mentioned briefly. Studies concerning a reversible opening of the blood-brain-barrier by HBO leading to an improved penetration of antibiotics with non-inflamed meninges are to be mentioned briefly as well.

We would like to state that HBO with intracranial abscesses, at present, should be applied only in combination and as a complement to other standard procedures of therapy (9); this means especially:
-neurosurgical approach (e.g. puncture, drainage, resection, all this depending on the individual situation);
-antibiotics;
-steroids.

The advantage of steroid application is a very controversial topic in the international literature (9), as well as several widely used antibiotic regimens, for example the combination of the bactericidal penicillins with the bacteriostatic substance chloramphenicole (11). Contrary to the other antibiotics, metronidazole with its reliable penetration capacity into the central nervous system, even with less inflamed meninges, is certainly invaluable. Nonetheless research and development of an even more efficient antibiotic access remains to be crucial (9), since quite a number of patients will not meet the requirements for safe surgical management. At this point hyperbaric oxygen will prove to be a promising component with major antibiotic capacity (6, 8, 10, 14). Its application has to be considered seriously with the following conditions:
-multiple abscesses;
-abscess in a deep or dominant location;
-early abscess stage with surgical intervention not being planned;
-poor patient condition;
-anaerobic findings from abscess material.

CONCLUSIONS

In spite of convincing theoretical facts as well as promising therapeutical results, animal experiments are urgent not to endorse the future benefit of HBO in the management of intracranial abscesses. All this is meant to lead to a transformation of the present "investigative indication" into a currently accepted one. It is of major importance to us, and this is meant to be a plea, to collect well-documented case reports together with the UHMS as much as possible in order to make a representative patient series. It's up to us all, to create a new "currently accepted indication" for HBO.

N.B.: Case reports demonstrated during the presentation will be published promptly in the Journal of Hyperbaric Oxygen:
    a) Epidural empyema due to frontal sinusitis;
    b) Parietal brain abscess combined with ischemic stroke due to pulmonary vascular malformation.

Bacterial Isolates	Brain Abscess	Subdural Empyema
Total No. of Cases	9	10
AEROBIC BACTERIA		
Gram positive cocci	4	1
Gram negative cocci	2	1
ANAEROBIC BACTERIA		
Gram positive cocci	9	7
Gram negative cocci	1	2
Gram positive bacilli	5	0
Gram negative bacilli	7	12
Subtotal Aerobes (N=8)	6	2
Subtotal Anaerobes (N=43)	22	21
Total No. of Bacteria	28	23

Figure 1. Bacterial isolates from 19 children with intracranial abscesses (11): for details see text. (Source: BROOK, J Neurosurg, 54 (4) 484-8, 1981)

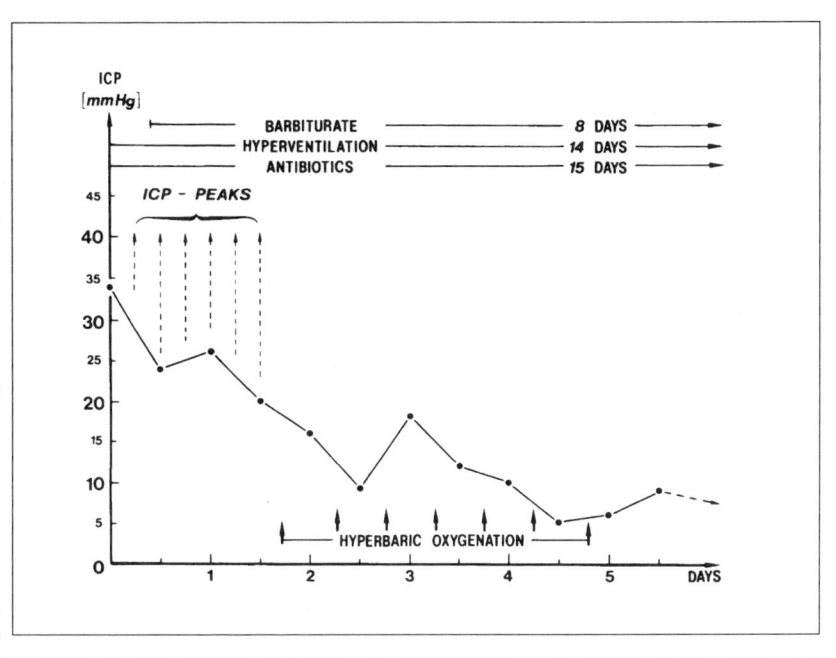

Figure 2. Development of the critically increased ICP in a patient with multiple brain abscesses (for detail see text).

REFERENCES

1. Brook I.: Bacteriology of intracranial abscess in children. J. Newrosur, 54 (4) 484-8, 1981
2. Dohrmann P.J., Elrick W.L.: Observations on brain abscesses. Review of 28 cases. Med J Aust, 2 (2) 81-3, 1982.
3. Gott U., Holbach K.H.: Hyperbare Sauerstofftherapie bei neurochirurgischen Patienten. Anasthesist, 18 (5) 139-45, 1969.
4. Harris L.F. et al.: Brain abscess: recent experience at a community hospital. South Med J, 78 (6) 704-7, 1985.
5. Heimbach R.D., Boerema I., Brummelkamp W.J., Wolfe W.G.: Current therapy of gas gangrene. In Davis J.C., Hunt T.K. (Eds.): Hyperbaric Oxygen Therapy. Undersea Medical Society, Bethesda, Md., 1977.
6. Hohn D.C.: Oxygen and leukocyte microbial killing. In Davis J.C., Hunt T.K. (Eds.): Hyperbaric Oxygen Therapy. Undersea Medical Society, Bethesda, Md., 1977.

7. Holbach K.H. et al.: Differentiation between reversible and irreversible post-strok changes in brain tissue: Its relevance for cerebrovascular surgery. Surg Neurol, 7, 325-31, 1977.
8. Irvin T.T. et al.: Hyperbaric oxygen in the treatment of infections by aerobic microorganisms. Lancet 1: 392-94, 1966.
9. Kaplan K.: Brain abscess. Med Clin North Am, 69 (2) 345-60, 1985.
10. Knighton D.R. et al.: Oxygen as an atibiotic. The effect of inspired oxygen on infections. Arch Sur, 119, 199-204, 1984.
11. Lampl L., Frey G., Miltner F.O., Worner U.: Multiple anaerobic brain abscesses - life saving hyperbaric oxygen therapy. In proceedings of the 9th International Congress on Hyperbaric Medicine, Undersea Medical Society, Bethesda, Md., 1986.
12. Ohta H. et al.: Intracranial pressure and hyperbaric oxygenation. In Proceedings of the 8th International Congress on Hyperbaric Medicine, Undersea Medical Society, Bethesda, Md., 1986.
13. Peirce E.C. II., Jacobsen J.H.II: Cerebral edema. In Davis J.C., Hunt T.K. (Eds.): Hyperbaric Oxygen Therapy, Undersea Medical Society, Bethesda, Md., 1977.
14. Schreiner A., Tonjun S., Digranes A.: Hyperbaric oxygen therapy in Bacteriodes infections. Acta Chir Scan, 140, 73-6, 1974.
15. Sukoff M.H., Ragatz R.E.: Hyperbaric oxygenation for the treatment of acute cerebral edema. Neurosurgery, 10, 29-38, 1982.

A preliminary report

Neurological effects of diving and decompression sickness

T. A. Anderson, R. G. Beran, C. W. Edmonds,
R. D. Green and M. Hodgson.

School of Underwater Medicine
Hmas Penguin
Balmoral
New South Wales 2091
Australia

ACKNOWLEDGEMENTS

The authors thank Monica Kleinman for assistance with psychometric assessment, Dr. V. Vignaendra for assistance with EEG assessment, and Dr. G. Shirtley for assistance with CT (brain) assessment.

KEY WORDS

Diving Decompression Sickness, Neurological Effects, Psychometric Assessment, CT Brain Scan, Electro-encephalography, Hyperbaric treatment

INTRODUCTION

Papers were presented at Kobe, Japan, Sep 86 (1) and at the ABC 35 Conference at Portsmouth, UK, Nov 86 (2) on behalf of the Royal Australian Navy School of Underwater Medicine. The papers reported findings and follow up details of an initially large group of air divers who had suffered decompression sickness and been treated at the School. At an early stage in the follow up of these divers, it became obvious that this could never be a study due to the almost exponential fall off of patients returning for regular review and assessment following discharge from treatment.

Such tendencies that were observed suggested that the type of psychometric testing that was being used was in all probability too gross in order to define minimal cerebral dysfunction which could have been due to decompression sickness. Since the last report in Nov 86, a further 14 divers have been reviewed at the one year stage following discharge. The tendencies previously described (1), (2), do not indicate the necessity for modification of these views and conclusions.

REVIEW AND UPDATE OF EXISTING DATA

87 divers with decompression sickness (DCS) were treated by the School of Underwater Medicine (SUM) between Feb 84 and Aug 86. In 6 cases clinical relief was not achieved at an early stage on a shallow (18 msw) Oxygen therapeutic regime. One of these cases was further compressed to 50 msw and decompressed on a long air table (RN 45). The other 5 were treated on a USN-1A (RAN modified) 30 msw variable-mix Oxy-Nitrogen regime. Daily short Oxygen treatments (RN 61) were administered for recurrence of perseverance of symptoms and signs until full resolution or until there had been no further improvement for 2 successive treatments.

Time span	One week	One month	Six months	One year
Follow-up review	Clinical	Clinical	Clinical	Clinical
	EEG	EEG	—	EEG
	CT Brain Scan	Ct Brain Scan	—	CT Brain Scan
	Psycho-Metric Testing	—	—	Psycho-Metric Testing

The clinical review was carried out independently by both an Underwater Medicine trained Medical Officer from SUM and by a Consultant Neurologist. All divers presenting for follow up at the 3 specific intervals were seen by the same Neurologist who also carried out and read the EEG. The EEGs were independently verified by a further Neurologist who was unaware of the clinical history.

CT scans were carried out by the same private radiological practice, but not necessarily reported by the same Radiologist, however they were independently verified by a further Radiologist who was unaware of the clinical history.

The psychometric evaluation was carried out by a Consultant Psychiatrist (fellow author CE), with training and specific interest in the psychometric evaluation of divers. The actual tests used were scored independently by a Clinical Psychologist who was unaware of the clinical history. The psychometric results were compared against the score of the individual's IQ as derived from the Australian Council of Education General Intelligence Test, the ACER (WL), standardized on the Australian population. The two specific psychometric tests used were the Benton Visual Retention Test (BVTR) and the Digit Symbol Test from the Weschler Adult Intelligence Scale (Revised).

The six-monthly clinical review was incorporated to reassess divers who had returned to diving having been passed medically fit to dive following full resolution of symptoms, signs and follow up investigation at the one month stage.

RESULTS

RECORDED ABNORMALITIES

Follow-up review	One week	One month	Six months	One year
EEG	22 (n=46)	8 (n=46)	—	3 (n=14)
CT SCAN	8 (n=40)	5 (n=40)	—	0 (n=4)
PSYCO-METRIC TESTING	20 (n=61)	—	—	3 (n=12)
CLINICAL	10 (n=46)	2 (n=46)	1 (n=23)	1 (n=14)

COMBINED ABNORMALITIES

Tests	One week	One month	One year
EEG CT PMT	0	—	0
EEG CT	8	5	0
CT PMT	0	—	0
EEG PMT	1	—	0

A view expressed by the Consultant Psychiatrist conducting the psychometric evaluation was that most subjects demonstrated evidence of a variable degree of psychological stress and anxiety which could well have a detrimental effect on their psychometric performance. Not only was this effect underestimated, but it was a factor which in itself was very difficult to estimate accurately. A possible extension from this was that 4 divers needed subsequent psychiatric treatment.

INTERIM CONCLUSIONS

The previously reported findings had indicated that further work in this field was necessary and that the existing investigations were probably too insensitive to elucidate subtle abnormalities. Electroencephalography appeared to have the most consistency, and abnormalities tended to resolve with time. The almost exponential fall off of divers presenting for follow-up assessment was a most unfortunate feature, but was ultimately beyond the control of the investigators.

Assessment of the pre-morbid state was one of the most difficult problems, and has never been satisfactorily evaluated with any degree of accuracy. The National Adult Reading Test (NART) (3) has been used in the assessment of the pre-morbid state. The test takes less than 10 minutes and involves recognizing and reading lists of increasingly complex words, currently in English only. Known limitations include variable correlation with intelligence testing, and biases of an educational, social and cultural nature. The test is therefore unlikely to be of use in assessment of the subject groups (see below), however its incorporation into the test battery could conceivably add to the knowledge and specificity of the test.

FUTURE STUDIES

It has long been suggested that diving might cause subtle neurological damage over a long period of time, particularly with Nitrogen as the inert gas in the mixture (4). Little work appears to have been conducted on this issue and it is of particular interest since air and Oxy-nitrogen mixture diving is the only diving currently in use in the Royal Australian Navy (other than Oxygen). In order to address this issue, a prospective cohort study had been initiated involving the neurological and psychometric comparison of three specific groups:

1. Divers with less than 5 years diving exposure.
2. Divers with more than 5 years diving exposure.
3. Matched non-divers.

A history of DCS would exclude divers from either group.

The study immediately ran into problems with the selection of both groups of divers. It had been considered that the only population of divers who would be available for the study and in whom DCS and a history of diving was reliably documented were divers from the Royal Australian Navy

Clearance Diving Branch. It was thought that this was a relatively "captive" group and that there would be much less likelihood of the progressive drop out of subject material that had been experienced in the work on DCS. The overwhelming majority of divers in the DCS work were civilian recreational divers, since during this period of time, RAN diving had yielded only 6 cases of DCS, all of whom were mild and responded rapidly with complete remission to treatment.

Following the call for volunteers for the study, none were forthcoming from the Clearance Diving Branch. On enquiry it transpired that the fear existed that if by means of investigation not normally used for the medical assessment of a diver's fitness, abnormal results were demonstrated, it might prejudice the diving career prospects of the individual. Counter views that the study was for the ultimate benefit of the diving community at large were relatively unheeded.

REVISED STUDY PROTOCOL

The parameters of the study were revised and it was decided to compare personnel joining the Clearance Diving Branch, who had either very limited or no diving exposure, with non-divers. The initial evaluation would be structured as part of their assessment of medical fitness to dive and would be re-evaluated at 5 year intervals. Matched pairs would be selected and similarly studied. The initial cohorts consist of all personnel (both Officers and Sailors) joining the Clearance Diving Branch during the next 3 years, ie a total of about 40 divers per year, which allowing for the inevitable few who do not complete the course, is expected to yield a total of over 100 divers. This group will be available for comparison with matched non-divers and each annual cohort of divers can be compared with the other two.

It has recently been suggested that the study could be extended to divers and non-divers with yet a third group, matched and selected from a non-Naval environment but with similar personality traits (probable risk takers) (5). Army parachutists, for instance would probably be ideal, however this has not yet been addressed in any detail.

CONTROL GROUP SELECTION

Control groups are matched on the following criteria:
Age
Sex
Social grouping
Personality traits
IQ assessment
General level of education

TESTING PRINCIPLES

It appears unlikely that the currently used non-invasive EEG procedures can be much improved over the expected duration of the study. Since electroencephalography is the only test procedure which has shown any degree of consistency in the previous work on DCS, it therefore forms and integral part of the test program.

The selection of psycho-metric testing must necessarily be governed by the following:
1. Capable of being carried out by a Department of Defense Psychologist with minimal additional training.
2. Sufficiently sensitive in order to detect minimal brain dysfunction.
3. Minimal subjective learning effect.
4. Restricted to a time duration which will avoid both subject and observer fatigue.
5. Sufficiently broad and searching to withstand critical analysis during and after the study period.

PSYCHO-METRIC TEST SELECTION

Psycho-metric testing is aimed at the evaluation of:
Psychomotor capability
Memory
Cortical function and processing

DISCUSSION ON SPECIFIC PSYCHO-METRIC TEST PROCEDURES

Although a limited amount of psycho-metric evaluation has been carried out on divers (4), (6), to date no studies are known which have spanned a diver's career. Air or Oxy-nitrogen mixed diving is thought to present a greater neuro-psychological hazard than Oxy-helium saturation diving (4). EEGs were not found to correlate with psycho-metric findings in deep diving. However the time frames involved have been weeks rather than years, and/or the numbers of subjects have been small, typically groups of 6 or 7 divers.

In using a similar testing system to that of the deep diving study (4), no psycho-metric deficit was demonstrated on a group of divers exposed to Central Nervous System (CNS) Oxygen Toxicity, (6). EEG recordings were not conducted in this work. Psycho-metric testing was carried out both pre- and post- dive. Some post-dive results which scored higher than pre-dive testing could conceivably have been influenced by a learning effect.

It appears to be generally accepted that the evaluation of minimal brain damage should include psycho-motor capability, memory, and cortical function and processing. There is not necessarily universal agreement as to how these concepts should be evaluated. In the design of this study, consultative advise has been obtained from the disciplines of psycho-metric evaluation of early dementia (7), (8), heavy metal exposure, neuro-toxicology and neuro-pharmacology (5).

General test of IQ, education and personality, such as the Otis, ACER (WL) and the Minnesota Multiphasic Personality Inventory, are seen as being important in the selection of matching subjects to controls. Subject performance on any given test and occasion will be modified by mood and emotional factors. At present this is difficult to quantify as is its effect on specific testing, nevertheless mood and emotion assessment should be recorded at each test session for subsequent analysis and integration with the overall test score. The Multiple Affect Adjective Check List is one such test, while the World Health Organization (WHO) neuro-toxicology test battery uses a Mood States Profile, (5).

Psycho-motor capability can be evaluated in a number of ways. Trail test are a simple and traditional procedure, but depend on fairly gross pathology to demonstrate any abnormality. The Perdue Peg Board, which tests visual-spacial-perception and psychomotor capability, involves all four dimensions, and appears to be sensitive.

Various adaptations of the Finger Oscillation Test exist, in which the finger either taps out a specific sequent, or taps out a maximum number of taps in a given time. The latter procedure is thought to depend significantly on the "physical fitness" or otherwise of the finger involved, and its mechanical integrity. It is therefore thought that the variant involving the tapped sequence is more of a discriminatory and useful test since it also involves a short term memory component.

A degree of overlap will invariably exist between psycho-motor capability anc cortical function and processing. At its most basic, Simple Reaction Time involves and "on/off" response to a stimulus which can be adapted to be either visual or audio. An extension of this is the Visual Flicker Fusion Test, currently used in the evaluation of heavy metal toxicology (5). The subject views a light flashing at a frequency of 70 Hz. At this frequency the light appears continuous. The frequency is gradually reduced until the subject signals that the light is observed to be flashing. In normality this would typically occur at a frequency of the order of 40 Hz.

Complex reaction time is more orientated towards cortical function and processing, and involves a stimulus requiring a signaled decision from a range of possible alternatives. Micro-computer software now exists for such testing, which has the advantage of standardizing the challenge, recording the response and scoring the test. In the evaluation of divers (and matched controls), a computer test is unlikely to cause problems, however in existing cases of minimal brain dysfunction from early stage Alzheimer's Disease, gazing at a green VDU screen was shown to increase the stress level of subjects, (7).

The Benton Visual Retention Test has 3 forms and requires the subject to memorize a geometrical shape which must subsequently be reproduced (pencil and paper) after a short time interval. It remains to be seen whether this test is too insensitive to reveal minimal brain damage over a long period of time, however it will be retained in the battery for the moment. The Simpson Memory Pictures (Shapes and Associated Tests) have been recently introduced (8), and appear more searching than the Benton. The Memory Pictures have 4 forms of cards with 12 simple pictures of common objects on each. A card is memorized over a given period of time and recalled verbally one hour later.

The test is standardized for a young population and differentiates normal from refined disorganization of memory and retrieval in the long and short term. The test can be made even more discriminatory by the requirement of picture-card recall at any given time frame greater that one hour.

Digit Symbol Modalities such as the Weschler Digit Symbol Test, involve the substitution of both words and figures for simple geometric shapes. This test encompasses both short term memory and cortical function and processing.

The investigation of memory function is completed by the Digit Span Test of the Weschler Memory Scale. This involves the subject repeating back to the observer an increasingly complex digit series, initially forwards and subsequently in reverse.

More neuro-physiological than neuro-psychological is the Brainstem Evoked Auditory Response. The test depends on accurate, sensitive and well calibrated equipment. It is capable of detecting the site of a deficit along the auditory pathway from the cochlea to the auditory cortex. The principle of the test dates back to the 1890s, when abnormalities in EEG waveforms were attributed to deficits in the hearing pathway. The test has been used in the investigation of demyelination and ischemia. Over a diver's career, a progressive, although usually slight, deterioration has been observed on many occasions. It has been suggested that divers may be exposed to greater auditory hazards than previously believed, since at some frequencies, the ear may be more susceptible to noise in water than air (9). Under these circumstances, this test could be a useful diagnostic procedure, however in the absence of an abnormal audiogram it is unlikely to demonstrate any abnormality.

Although most of these tests are standardized, the concept of standardization exists for comparison with an individual's absolute score, possibly modified by existing or reasonably expected assessments of IQ and education. In this particular study, standardization assumes less importance, since the previous score of the study group forms the standard for subsequent assessment provided the same test protocol is used.

CONCLUSION

A variable degree of neurological dysfunction may be associated with air and Oxy-nitrogen mixture diving. Although EEG abnormalities have been reported in association with DCS, at a prevalence greater than might reasonable by expected in the normal population, concurrently conducted psycho-metric evaluation (Benton VRT and Weschler Digit Symbol Test) did not correlate either with each other or with the EEG findings. Such testing is now thought to have been too insensitive to elucidate any minimal brain damage which might conceivably have been present, either transient or permanent. CT scan correlated with EEG findings in only a small minority of cases, and are thought not to be of routine diagnostic or epidemiological use in the investigation of diving and DCS. A prospective cohort study of Royal Australian Navy Clearance Divers, compared with non-divers and possibly a third group of "risk takers" (or similarly structured study) is though to be the only way to address the question of the possibility of minimal brain damage due to long term exposure to air of Oxy-nitrogen diving. This study should be programmed to run for 20 years (the reasonably expected maximum duration of a military diving career), with individual and group re-assessment at 5 yearly intervals. These findings should be reported and published as they become available. Assessments should include electroencephalography and a sufficiently detailed and sensitive battery of psycho-metric tests aimed at the demonstration or otherwise of minimal and subtle brain dysfunction.

REFERENCES

1. Gorman D.F., Edmonds D.W., Parsons D.W., Beran R.G., Anderson T.A., Green R.D., Loxton M.J., Dillon T.A. The Neurological Sequelae of Decompression Sickness: A Clinical Report. Ninth International Symposium on Hyperbaric Physiology. Kobe, Japan, Sep 86.
2. Anderson T.A., Beran R.G., Dillon T.A., Green R.D., Loxton M.J., Gorman D.F., Parsons D.W., Edmonds C.E. Neurological Assessment in Decompression Sickness: A Clinical Report. ABC 35 Conference, Portsmouth, UK, Nov 86.
3. Nelson H.E., O'Connell A. Dementia: The Estimation of Pre-morbid Levels Using the new Adult Reading Test. Cortex, 14, 234-244, 1978.
4. McIver N.K.I. (Ed). Various Approaches to Neuro-psychological Evaluation of Deep Divers. European Undersea Biomedical Society and Norwegian Petroleum Directorate Workshop, Stavager. 14-16 Nov 83.

5. Williamson, Ann (PhD), New South Wales Dept of Industrial Relations (Occupational Health). Neuro-Psychological Testing in Heavy Metal Toxicology. Personal Communication, Feb 87.
6. Curley M.D., Robin G.J., Acute CNS Oxygen Toxicity and Diver Health. ABC 35 Conference, Portsmouth UK, Nov 86.
7. Drummond P. (PhD). Neuro-psychology Unit, Repatriation General Hospital, Concord, Sydney. Neuro-psychological Testing in Early Dementia. personal communication, Feb 87.
8. Simpson F. (PhD). Neuro-psychology Unit, Repatriation General Hospital, Concord, Sydney. Neuro-psychological Testing in Early Dementia. Personal Communication, Feb 87.
9. Smith R.F., Research on Hearing Conservation Standards for US Navy Divers. ABC 35 Conference Nov 86.

Changes of thromboxane A2 and prostacyclin in rabbits suffering from decompression sickness

J. Zhang, Supervisor: Prof. G. T. Ni

Department of Naval Medicine, Second Military Medical University, Shanghai, China

It has been recognized that victims of decompression sickness (DCS) have some manifestations of disturbance of respiratory and circulatory systems. Thromboxane A_2 (TxA_2) has a contraction effect on the vascular and the tracheobronchial smooth muscle and has an accelerating effect on platelet aggregation, whereas prostacyclin ($OPGI_2$) has a relaxation effect on the vascular and the tracheobronchial smooth muscle and has an anti-platelet aggregation effect (1). However, little evidence is available regarding the roles of TxA_2 and PGI_2 in DCS. As a step toward identifying the roles, we evaluated the values of plasma thromboxane B_2 (TxB_2) and 6-keto-PGF_1 (the stable respective metabolites of TxA_2 and PGI_2) in experimental DCS. The prophylactic effect of indomethacin (cyclo-oxygenase inhibitor) on acute DCS was also investigated.

MATERIALS AND METHODS

Animal preparation. Male, New Zealand white rabbits (weighing 1.85 to 2.5 kg) were divided into three groups: adequate decompression group (group I), inadequate decompression group (group II) and indomethacin-treated group (group III). A catheter was inserted into the right atrium of each animal through an external jugular vein for a blood sampling. And the catheter was filled with heparinized saline, which was replaced every 12 hours. Hairs covering the cardial area skin were shaven for Doppler bubble detection and a subsequent tape recording. Compression-decompression treatment was performed in an animal compression chamber after 3-6 days of operation.

Drug administration. Immediately before use, indomethacin was dissolved in a minimum volume of 0.5 N NaOH and diluted to the desired concentration (5mg/ml) with phosphate buffer (0.2 M, pH 7.4). It was slowly given intravenously 60 min before the compression to deliver a dose of 10 mg/kg to the group III.

DCS in rabbits. In the group I the chamber was compressed with air to a pressure of 709 kpa at a rate of 303 kpa/min. After a bottom time of

30 min, the chamber was decompressed to 12 m within 5 min and then gradually decompressed according tot he following schedule (one minute between stops).

Depth of stop (m)	12	9	6	3
Duration of stoppage (min)	4	8	10	15

In the group II the chamber was decompressed at a rate of 202 kpa/min to the surface after a bottom time of 30 min. While in the group III, the decompression was finished within 1.5 min.
Measurement of TxB2 and 6-keto-PGF12. Time of blood sampling.

	pre-compression		post-decompression		
Group I	-60		20		90
Group II	-60		20	60	180
Group III	-60	-20	20		90

Every time, 2.5 ml blood was obtained from the catheter by using a syringe filled with 0.1 ml saline containing heparin and indomethacin. The blood samples were put into ice-cooled tubes and were centrifuged at 1000 g for 10 min. The supernatant was acidified to pH 3.5-4.0 (HCL), extracted with 5 ml either from petroleum. The sediment was again extracted twice with 5 ml ethyl acetate, which was then removed by evaporation under a stream of nitrogen. The dried extract was stored at -20°C until their determination by RIA. (in dying animals the blood sampling had been performed before the respiration completely ceased).

Doppler ultrasonic bubble detector was used and signals were recorded before the blood sampling.

RESULTS

In the group II, ten of twenty-three rabbits died of DCS within 45 min after the decompression, while the rest showed various degree of signs of DCS (respiratory distress, bends or only vasoconstriction of ear blood vessels). Signals of Doppler ultrasound detected were grade 2 or grade 3 in survivors and grade 3 or grade 4 in dying animals. In the group I and group III, none of them showed any signs of DCS except two rabbits of group III had a minor and transient vasoconstriction of ear blood vessels. Doppler ultrasound was grade 0 or grade 1 in the former and grade 2 or grade 3 in the latter.

The levels of TxB2 and 6-keto-PGF1 are shown in table 1 and 2. In rabbits which were dying of DCS, TxB2 levels were higher than those of the pre-compression controls ($P<0.01$). While in the survivors they were decreased at 20 min and restored at 180 min after decompression ($P<0.01$). No significant change was observed in the group I. In group II TxB2 levels decreased significantly after the administration of indomethacin and no statistic significance were obtained between, before and after the compression decompression treatment. 6-keto-PGF1 levels were also increased in animals dying of DCS (P<0.01). No statistic significance was obtained in the survivors of group II and in the group I.

The animals which died and were shown in the table 1 were dead between 18 min and 22 min, the three others were dead between 40 min and 45 min in which TxB2 and 6-keto-PGF1 levels were increased progressively. In the survivors of group II, blood samples of three animals were given up because the tubes were crashed during centrifugation.

Table 2. Values of Plasma TxB2 in Group III

Before Injection -60	Before Compression -20	After Decompression to the surface		
		20	90	(min)
479.16** (±141.06)	261.80 (±53.90)	268.74 (±68.80)	235.86 (±38.48)	

(pg/ml, mean ± SD, n=9, **: P<0.01)

DISCUSSION

Although from the present study we can not identify the source of TxA2 and PGI2 synthesis in rabbits (platelet, leukocyte or other parts of the body), however, it is found that a population of normal rabbits can be divided into two groups, sensitive and insensitive, depending on the increase of TxB2 levels or not and a subsequent death or not. Ward et al (2) reported that if the rabbits are sensitive to complement activation at the plasma-air or serum-air interface, they lead to polymorphonuclear leukocyte aggregation. Intravascular complement activation may result in TxA2 production, pulmonary hypertension, hypoxemia and increased lung vascular permeability (3). The increase of tracheal and pulmonary artery blood pressure induced by room air infusion were suppressed significantly by premedication of TxA2 synthetase inhibitors (4). Though the precise role of arachidonic acid cascade in DCS is far from clear, it is reasonable to expect that cyclo-oxygen-ase inhibitors such as indomethacin could be useful drugs for the prevention of DCS.

Table 1. Values of Plasma TxB$_2$ and 6-keto-PGF1$_{xxx}$

	Animals	Before compression -60	20	After decompression to the surface 60	90	180 (min)
TxB$_2$ (pg/ml)	Group I (n=10)	421.24 (±223.11)	442.62 (±146.75)		499.70 (±181.91)	
	Group II					
	Dying animals (n=7)	531.20 (±48.81)	880.93** (±179.91)			
	Survivors (n=10)	632.36 (±327.06)	453.64** (±210.54)	474.77 (±200.66)		607.21 (±309.64)
6-keto-PGF$_1$XXX (pg/ml)	Group I (n=9)	439.88	471.10 (±175.63)	(±147.15)	447.54	(±218.52)
	Group II					
	Dying animals (n=7)	567.66 (±108.51)	1315.34** (±578.58)			
	Survivors (n=10)	571.15 (±254.86)	528.02 (±199.43)	601.28 (±293.73)		566.53 (±376.69)

REFERENCES

1. Sun QW: Effects of arachidonic acid metabolites on the lung. Progress in Physiological Sciences. 17: 129-133, 1986.
2. War CA, et al: Activation of complement at plasma-air or serum-air interface of rabbits. J. Appl. Physiol. 60: 1651-1658, 1986.
3. Gee MH, et al: Thromboxane as a mediator of pulmonary dysfunction during intravascular complement activation in sheep. Am. Rev. Respir. Dis. 133: 269-273, 1986.
4. Ishihara Y, et al: Effect of thromboxane synthetase inhibitors (OKY-046, OKY-1580) on experimentally induced air embolism in anesthetized dogs. Prostaglandins Leukotrienes Med. 21: 197-206, 1986.

The use and abuse of oxygen in Australian diving

Carl Edmonds

Dr Carl Edmonds, MB, BS, MRCP (Lond), FRACP, FACOM, DipDHM, FRANZCP Director, Diving Medical Centre, Cremorne, 2090, AUSTRALIA

REVIEW

Because I have been involved in Australian diving medicine over the last two decades, I have restricted my observations on the use of oxygen (O_2) to that period.

On August 10, 1967, two navy divers using O_2 sets, died during a training manoeuvre. The rumors were rife regarding Russian submarines, shark attack, desertion whilst on duty, and some more exotic explanations. Then, their bodies were found. Her Majesty's Coroner and the Naval Boards of Inquiry, based on the advice of experts, attributed the tragedies to "Shallow Water Blackout" or O_2 Syncope.

Just after that episode, I took over the Royal Australian Navy School of Underwater Medicine. It was essential, both for morale and for future safety of divers, that a solution and prevention of the problem be found.

Reviewing the literature on O_2 diving revealed that "shallow water blackout" [1] was described in 1944 by Barlow and MacIntosh at the RNPL, and was attributed to CO_2 toxicity in the rebreathing sets.

Professor Donald, in brilliant and extensive experiments, in 1945 [2] described the neurological toxicity, especially convulsions, with O_2 pressures >2 ATA. There were two interesting individual cases in his series who lost consciousness without an apparent convulsion.

Divers continued to suffer a high incidence of loss of consciousness at depths which did not produce convulsions. Sir Stanley Miles in 1957 [3], based loosely on the work of Donald, coined the term "O_2 syncope" for a form of O_2 poisoning that was aggravated by a plethora of others factors and caused unconsciousness, and therefore death, in many cases.

The improvements in diving equipment resulted in both Donald and Miles dismissing CO_2 as a factor because of the greater absorbent abilities in the new sets.

Thus, by 1967, we were confronted and confounded by a poorly defined diagnosis of "O_2 syncope", which occurred in divers at 30 foot or less using 100% O_2. There was no way of predicting which divers would be affected.

Using an embarrassingly simple approach (4,5) we conducted a series of dives to identify this disorder and determine exactly what was the major factor likely to predispose to it.

There were three divers, myself and two others, who performed a series of dives replicating the very demanding dive profile responsible for the deaths of the navy divers. There were two modifications.

1. They would be performed in daylight.
2. There was a medical support team attending each diver.

Three totally different diving sets were used:-

a. O_2 rebreathing set.
b. Scuba filled with 100% O_2.
c. Scuba filled with air.

This way, if an incident did occur, it would be possible to determine whether it was more related to the rebreathing equipment, O_2 as such, or the diving environment. We rotated the equipment with each trial.

Under these circumstances, within 60 minutes, we were able to produce a partial or total loss of consciousness in one of the three divers. It always occurred in the diver using the rebreathing set. It never occurred in the divers using either Scuba O_2, or Scuba air.

Not only that, but after dragging the unconscious subject from the water and resuscitating him, we placed his equipment on a new, fit healthy diver, and he would last only another 5 - 10 minutes.

Sophistication in the form of respiratory gas analysis, and replacing 100% O_2 with O_2 mixtures, verified that the unconsciousness in our divers had nothing to do with O_2. We demonstrated the same aetiology as Barlow and MacIntosh had 25 years previously, CO_2 toxicity.

Such experiments nowadays would have some difficulty passing the Ethics Committee.

Even with many of the modern rebreathing sets, the absorbent systems have not improved significantly to be safe for the use with maximal underwater exertion, for the alleged duration of most of the sets.

We learned a valuable lesson from these experiments. At depths of 30 foot or less, that O_2 possibly did not deserve its awesome reputation as a neurological toxin.

OXYGEN IN TREATMENT

In Australia during the late 1960s, because we were not obtaining ideal results with serious cases of decompression sickness (DCS) on conventional treatment tables, we decided to be more flexible in tailoring individual treatment to each case. The large number of patients allowed us repeatedly to observe the clinical results and modify our approaches.

Over the five years, 1967-1972, (6), we recompressed the patients to whatever depth significantly relieved the symptoms, and then gave the highest possible O_2 mixture, calculated at each depth to avoid both neurological and respiratory toxicity. These are now referred to as the "Australian Experimental Tables". They are not suitable for routine use, but are valuable to experienced therapists.

It is virtually impossible to produce valid comparisons of treatment tables, because of the great variety of both symptomatology of DCS and the expertise of the therapists. Nevertheless, in 1975 (7) the results were collated on 115 cases of DCS, treated in Australia and Singapore and the results were better with the Australian than with the conventional tables. The variable were too great to claim that this was "proven". The Australian tables were used only by those therapists who were already very experienced and this would have weighed results in their favor.

Four interesting developments (6,8) eventuated from this work.

Firstly, the use of 100% O_2 on the surface instead of recompression therapy. Some patients with minor or musculo-skeletal DCS presented very late (e.g. the following day), well after tissue gases would have equilibrated. These patients often responded to the use of 100% O_2 on the surface, over a period of 4-8 hours.

Another spin-off from the Australian tables was the use of 100% O_2 immediately after successful recompression therapy. Even in circumstances in which the symptoms had already recurred, the use of O_2 on the surface often removed them. In some cases the surface O_2 could be titrated against the patients symptomatology. Certainly the use of O_2, after the recompression therapy, reduced the need for subsequent recompressions.

Another development was the frequent use of 100% O_2 at nine meters, simulating the tables used by caisson physicians of yesteryear. In less severe cases the nine meter O2 table, without any air breaks, avoided some of the problems of the 19 meter tables - such problems as the redevelopment of symptoms during or immediately following the air breaks, and the occasional O_2 convulsion.

The most contentious aspect of the Australian experimental tables was the extension of this shallow O_2 table to the underwater environment.

In the South Pacific region, around the Australian area, there is a great paucity of recompression chambers, and of experienced personnel to use them. In the decade from 1967 onwards, the Navy was obligated to treat vast numbers of civilian divers. We had no adequate portable chambers, and had only one very restricted multi man chamber based in Sydney, with a catchment area that included countries such as Papua New Guinea, the Solomon Islands, Narau, Fiji, New Caledonia and the New Hebrides.

There was sometimes a lapse of 12-24 hours between the patient getting DCS and receiving treatment. The cost in time and money and the commitment of service facilities and aircraft, made treatment of minor cases impracticable. The delays made serious cases worse.

The underwater O_2 treatment was introduced to contend with these difficulties. The equipment was simple to organize and allowed divers to go to nine meters and gradually ascend (decompress) on O_2, over the period of two to three hours.

The underwater O_2 was used in treating mild cases which would otherwise not receive treatment, and also while arranging transport for some serious cases to Sydney. The underwater O_2 (followed by O_2 on the surface) often resulted in the transport not subsequently being required.

Initially the underwater O_2 was very contentious, and for that reason it was little publicized. Most of the criticisms came from people who had not carefully examined the procedure, or who had not calculated the UPTDs, and they were almost always from groups which had extensive and expensive hyperbaric facilities available to them.

It has now acquired the inevitable trappings of acceptability. I have been accused of purloining it from the French, and admonished by the Italians and Hawaiians for not going deeper and longer; it has been used from the Equator to the Antarctic; it was given an official number in the Australian Diving Manual in 1975.; it is included (with modifications that concern me) in the latest U.S. Navy Diving Manual. With each modification, a simple treatment is becoming more complex.

MISCELLANEOUS

The use of 100% O_2 on the surface, as a first aid measure and during transport, is nowadays accepted in cases of decompression sickness, barotraumas with gas pockets, and in near-drowning.

When I worked in the Flying Doctor Service, if a patient developed a spontaneous pneumothorax and it was impossible to reach him to do a thoracentesis, we used 100% O_2 to reduce the volume of the pneumothorax. In diving accidents, especially when the pneumothorax is not life threatening, we have used this same technique. It is even more effective in removing the gas from mediastinal emphysema within a few hours.

An interesting variation of this, is with orbital emphysema (8). A number of cases have been seen when divers injured the nasal bones (lamina papyracea), usually from playing football or fighting. Usually asymptomatic, there is then a potential opening between the nose and the orbit. Performing the Valsalva forces air into the orbit. The first such case we had caused great confusion as the diver had performed a Valsalva at about 30 feet, and suddenly his eye closed. As he ascended the gas expanded, and on the surface it was impossible to open the eyelids for examination. While transporting him to the chamber we administered 100% 02, and by the time he reached the chamber enough air had dissipated from the orbit to allow him to open his eye a little and for us to examine it. The ideal treatment for such cases would be the compression to nine meters with 100% O_2.

The major problem with divers administering O_2 for first aid, is a lack of familiarity with resuscitation equipment.

Adaptors were developed which allowed divers to use O_2 cylinders and obtain 100% O_2 through a diving regulator. The first of these, to my knowledge, was the Manly adaptor which was produced in 1970 by John Manly in the Royal Australian Navy.

A civilian counterpart of this was developed and promoted in 1983 by Bob Sands, and enthusiastic entrepreneur and dive instructor, north of Sydney. The BENDEEZ allowed drivers to breathe O_2 via Scuba regulators, from commercial or medical O_2 cylinders and the OXIVIVA. Most well operated dive boats carry these facilities now and there have been a number of cases in which the BENDEEZ appeared to be of great value. I understand that the system is being made available in North America.

In 1985 a survey was done on the abalone divers in Australia (9). These divers have excessive hyperbaric exposures. According to the conventional U.S. Navy tables, 58% of the divers routinely employed a dive profile which required decompression, but which was omitted.

Because of the prevalence of DCS, one quarter of the divers over the last few years use O_2 and 13.2% use it underwater, either for treatment or prevention. Some use it in excess of 30 feet and have experienced O_2 toxicity in depths greater that 60 feet. They do not just hang on a line decompressing, they use the O_2 time to collect more abalone!

This regular use of O_2 underwater may produce interesting data in the years to come, but I hope not.

It is important to reiterate that I have summarized some way in which O_2 has been used in Australian diving over the last 20 years. I have not attempted moral or other judgements regarding its value, and I have not attempted to condone or support it. I have merely reported on the practices.

REFERENCES

1. Barlow, H.B. and MacIntosh F.C. (1944) Shallow Water Black-out. MRC Report RNP 44-125.
2. Donald, K.W. (1946). Oxygen Poisoning in Man. AEDU Report No. 16.
3. Miles, S. (1957). Oxygen Syncope. MRC Report. RNP 57-880.
4. Edmonds, C. (1968). Shallow Water Blackout. Project 8-68 School of Underwater Medicine, RAN.
5. Edmonds, C. (1968). The Hypercanoeic Syndrome. Project 2-86. School of Underwater Medicine Report, RAN.
6. Edmons, C., Lowry, C. and Pennefather, J. (1976) <u>Diving and Subaquatic Medicine</u>. 1st Edition. Diving Medical Centre Publications, Cremore, 2080, Australia.
7. How, J., West D. and Edmonds, C. (1976) Decompression Sickness in Diving. Singapore Med. J. 17(2); 92-97.
8. Edmonds, C., Lowry, C.J. and Pennefather, J. (1981) <u>Diving and Subaquatic Medicine</u>. 2nd Edition. Diving Medical Centre Publication, Cremore, 2080, Australia.
9. Edmonds, C. (1986) <u>The Abalone Diver</u>. National Safety Council Publication, Morwell, Victoria.

Effects of Temperature on Oxygen Toxicity in Rats at Pressures to 6 ATA.

P. B. Bennett and K. E. Pinkerton

F.G. Hall Laboratory
Duke Medical Center
Durham, North Carolina 27710
and Anatomy Department
University of California
Davis, California 95616, USA

When breathing 100% oxygen at increased pressures, signs and symptoms of toxicity depend on both the pressure and the time at pressure (1). In man the primary central nervous system (CNS) effect is the well known oxygen seizure which may occur usually at pressures in excess of 3 ATA often with out prodromal signs or symptoms but is accompanied by classical seizure activity in the electroencephalogram. Should the exposure to oxygen continue then further convulsions and death may result.

At 2 ATA and lower pressures, CNS toxicity is not the problem but the emphasis switches to the lung. Oxygen toxicity of the lung involves destruction of both capillary endothelium and alveolar endothelium, alveolar cell hyperplasia, edema, hemorrhage, arterial thickening and hyalinization, fall in vital capacity, hypoxemia and death (1).

Although much research has been done on the mechanism of oxygen toxicity, its true mechanism remains elusive and sometimes controversial. Thus to make diving safer the problem of oxygen toxicity is evaded by keeping the oxygen pressure below the limits necessary for the onset of toxicity at normal body temperatures. For the U.S. Navy this means 25 ft (1.8 ATA).

As a consequence many attempts also have been made to modify oxygen tolerance (3-6) by utilizing antioxidants and oxidants, hormonal factors, metabolic and nutritional factors, effects of carbon dioxide, inert gas effects and adaptation (1).

Remarkably little work, however, has been done on the direct effects of temperature per se, although it has been examined indirectly by studies of increased or decreased metabolic activity. In 1949, Grossman and Penrod (7) suggested that hypothermia offered a means of relating general metabolic level to high oxygen toxicity in the absence of other factors such as drugs or anesthesia. They cooled rats to rectal temperature of 20°, 25°, and 30°C at 5.2 or 5.8 ATS for 1 hour. A strong correlation was observed between survival and metabolic rate but the paper gives no data on the cause of death, lung pathology, etc. and the time was restricted to 1 hour at between 5-6 ATS. Further the animals were cooled prior to placing in the chamber and compression, so the actual temperature is unclear at pressure and there were many other flaws in the study.

More recently Kovatchich (8) studied a variety of conditions affecting metabolism that increase oxygen toxicity in the brain slices. All of these had one common factor in that they increased the respiratory rate of the brain tissue. Conversely other conditions including cooling the in vitro medium from 37° to 32° and reduced respiratory rate made the brain tissue less sensitive to oxygen at pressures of 5 to 10 ATS.

There are only a few other studies including Puglia, Glauser and Glauser (9) in 1974 on the fall of core temperature response as a prelude to hyperbaric oxygen convulsions and, in connection with the space program preflight studies for Apollo 7, on the tolerance of pocket mice to oxygen and heat on the brain (10) and lung (11) at pressures of only 8, 10 or 12 psi for 7 days. No unusual effects were noted.

The research to be described therefore sought to examine the CNS and pulmonary effects of exposure of rats to increased pressures of oxygen up to 6 ATA while exposed to either cold, normal or hot environmental temperatures.

METHODS

Groups of 12 male Sprague-Dawley rats (260 - 320 grams) were exposed, 4 at a time, to 100% oxygen at pressures of 1, 3 and 6 ATA at 9.2 m/min and at temperatures of 8, 25 or 37°C. For one of the four rats, skin temperature was measured over the lateral aspect of the flank just caudal to the rib cage, and core temperature from a rectal probe (accuracy ±/- 0.5°C) while gently restrained in a holding sleeve. Exposures to 1 and 3 ATA were for 6 hrs but at 6 ATA were abbreviated to 40 mins due to convulsions. Pulmonary toxicity was determined by a numerical scale of changes in lung morphology, with 0 being no pathology and 4 extensive perivascular cuffing of all vessels accompanied by hemorrhage and edema in the alveoli. In addition, an edema ration was devised to measure the thickness of the cuffs surrounding the pulmonary vessels. This expressed the cuff to vessel area as an estimate of the relative degree of fluid accumulation surrounding each vessel normalized to vessel size using a digitizer interfaced to a computer.

All exposures were done in a 1.33 cubic meter Bethlehem hyperbaric chamber. The temperature was regulated with a heating and cooling system contained within the design of the chamber. Each experiment was done with four animals placed in partitioned compartments in an airtight polycarbonate box in the chamber. The weight of each animal was recorded. Prior to pressurization of the chamber, the box was purged with oxygen and the concentration of oxygen and carbon dioxide was determined. In all cases the oxygen concentration was greater than 98.5% and the carbon dioxide concentration less that 0.15%. During the course of the experiment oxygen and carbon dioxide concentrations were again measured and found to be similar to those prior to pressurization. Oxygen flow through the chamber was maintained at 10 - 15 liters per minute.

RESULTS

Skin and Core Temperature of the Rats

At 1 ATA the skin and core temperatures decreased from 1° to 3° over the six hour period of exposure to oxygen (Fig. 1). However, monitored animals exposed to 37°C at 1 ATA were unable to tolerate exposure for 6 hours. The combined stress of oxygen and restraint were sufficient to cause death even in the absence of hyperbaric conditions. Further, exposure to 6 ATA of oxygen was too short at this pressure to conclusively demonstrate a significant temperature effect.

The most striking effects of different environmental temperatures were noted in exposures to 3 ATA of oxygen (Fit 2). This led to the loss of body temperature regulation especially in animals exposed to cold temperatures. On the other hand, animals exposed to warmer temperatures (i.e., 25 and 37°C) had a higher mortality rate which was preceded by a 5 to 7 degree C increase in skin and core body temperatures prior to death (Fig. 3).

Central Nervous System Toxicity

Convulsions were most evident at 6 ATA only, with times ranging from 10 to 33 mins.

An interesting finding was that the onset of seizures was not sufficient to induce pathology in the lungs. Such changes in lung morphology required an additional exposure of 4 to 8 mins at hyperbaric oxygen before this occurred (Fig. 3).

The rats exposed to 6 ATA at 37°C showed a mean convulsion time of 19.3 ± 3.5 mins compared to 25 ± 6.4 mins for animals at 25°C and 20.5 ± 4.3 mins for those at 8°C. Only the hot animals results were statistically significant using the Bartlett test for homogeneity of variance (Table 1).

Seizure activity at 3 ATA of oxygen was infrequently observed. However, during the fourth hour of exposure labored breathing was noted indicative of pulmonary changes.

Pulmonary Changes

Changes in the lungs were most sever and occurred in the shortest period of time following oxygen exposure at 6 ATA compared to exposures at 1 and 3 ATA. The most striking and sever changes in the lungs was fulminant pulmonary edema noted grossly as heavy, hemorrhagic lungs which microscopically showed the flooding of alveoli with proteinous, eosinophilic fluid and blood and prominent accumulations of fluid and blood in the interstitial space surrounding the pulmonary vasculature. These changes in the degree of edema were fairly rapid and at 6 ATA of oxygen the difference between no perivascular cuffing and marked cuffing was the matter of a few additional minutes of maintaining exposure conditions following the onset of seizures.

It was found that perivascular cuffing was most prominent along the arterial and venous vessels accompanying the major airway entering the lobe with vascular cuffing along the branches of these vessels. Cuffing appeared more prominenet in the hilar region and around arterial vessels compared to veins (Table 2).

Although only animals which survived the exposure were evaluated it was noted that animals which died had heavy hemorrhagic lungs with striking perivascular ciffing and fluid accumularion in alveolar spaces. Therefore the higher mortality rates at 37°C compared to 8°C are most likely due to a result of severe compromised lung function as a result of pulmonary oxygen toxicity.

Discussion and Conclusions

It is evident that the role of temperature on oxygen toxicity is complex. However, from a mortality point of view, animals exposed to HBO at 37°C were much more severely affected. This is shown both by the higher mortality and the shorter time to convulsions. Since the mortality was primarily due to massive pulmonary problems it may be concluded that both neurological and pulmonary oxygen toxicity are enhanced by high temperatures.

At cold temperatures, on the other hand, the mortality is if anything less severe than in animals at normal temperatures but these results are influenced by the inability of the animals to maintain thermal equilibrium which led to hypothermia.

Further, these results confirm earlier investigators' findings that pulmonary edema following exposure to hyperbaric oxygen is due to central nervous system disturbances resulting in massive sympathetic discharge and central pooling of blood into the pulmonary circulation (13). We have found too that persistent exposure of the brain to HBO is associated with marked perivascular cuffing in the lungs. This cuffing is more pronounced for arterial vessels compared to venous vessels.

These results could have important ramifications to military individuals and patients in relation to the environmental temperature when they are exposed to HBO.

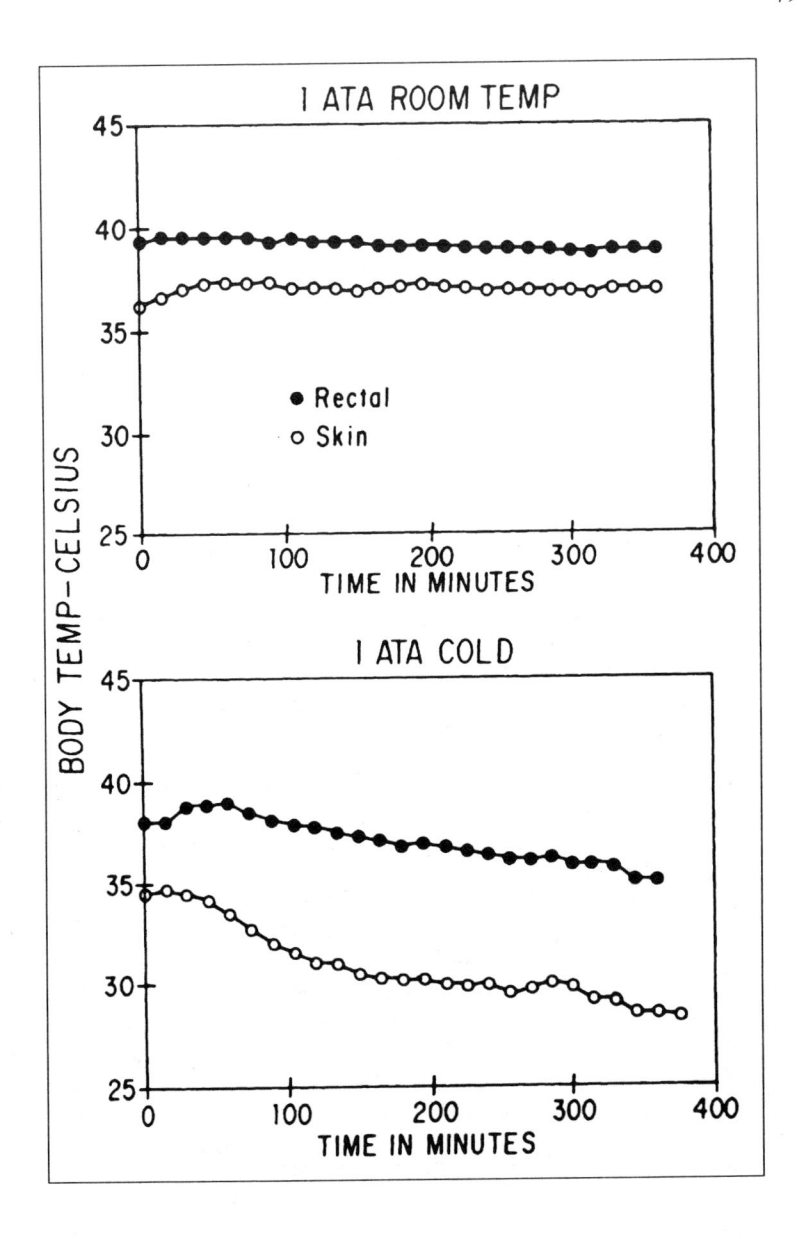

Figure 1. Skin (lower line) and core (upper line) temperatures of rates exposed to 1 ATA oxygen at room temperature and at 8oC over 6 hours. A decrease opf 1-3oC was noted especially in the cold.

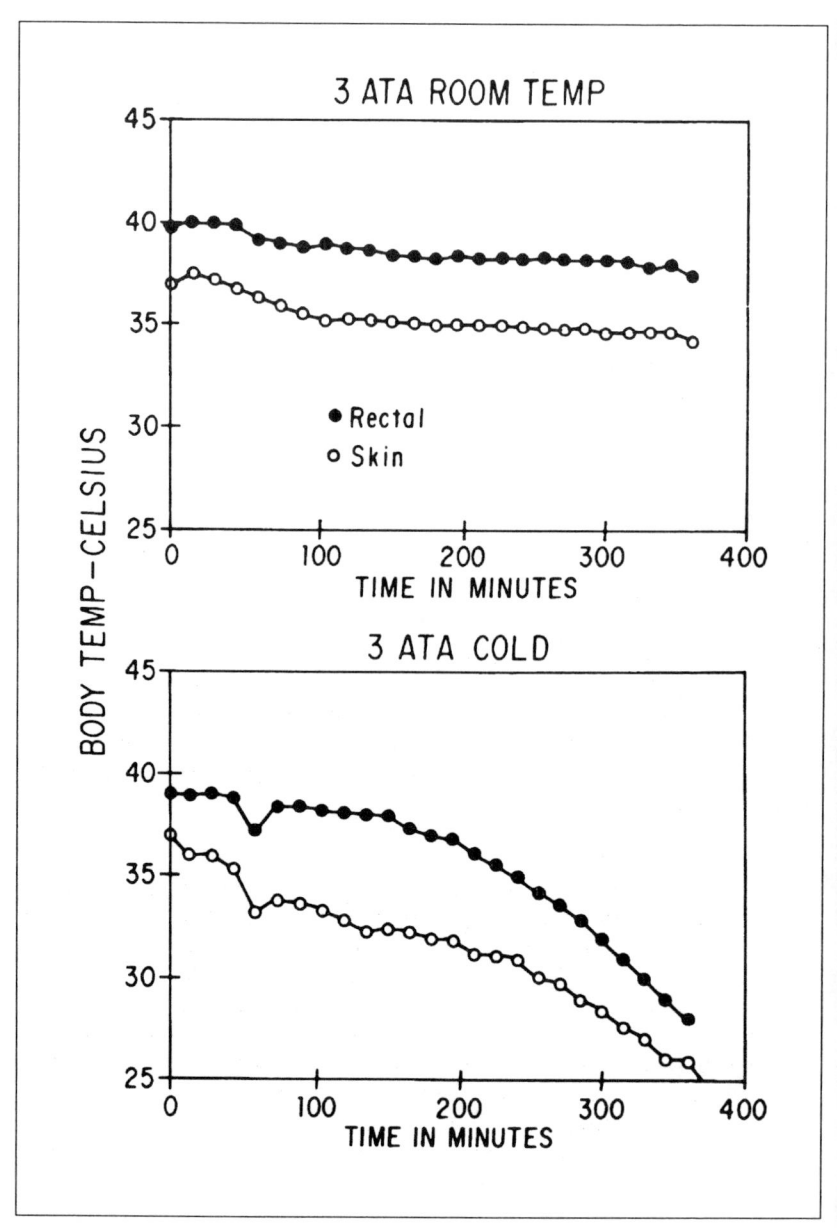

Figure 2. Skin (lower line) and core (upper line) temperatures of rats exposed to 3 ATA at room temperature and at 8°C over 6 hours. A loss of temperature regulation occurred at about 2 hours at 3 ATA oxygen.

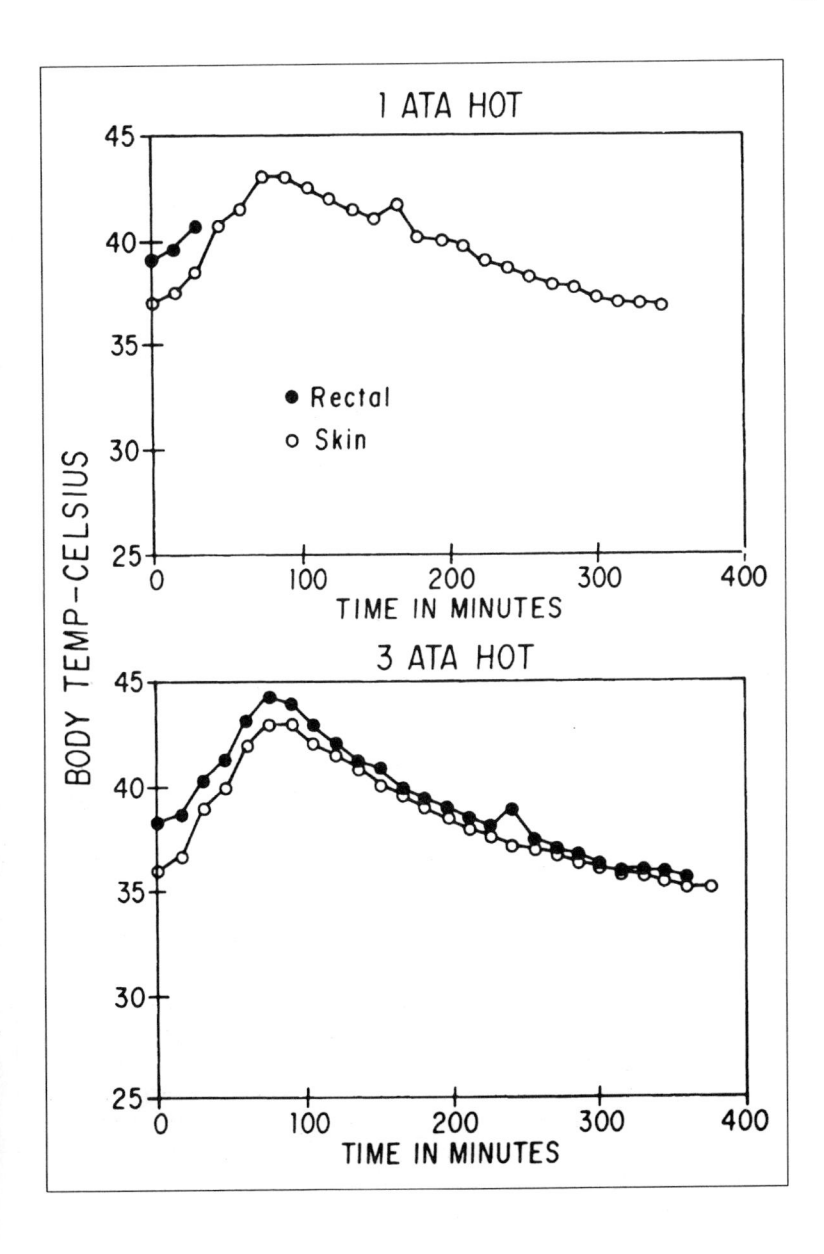

Figure 3. Skin (lower line) and core (upper line) temperatures of rats exposed to 1 ATA and 3 ATA at 37°C. Note increase in rectal and skin temperatures

Table 1. Response of Rats to Hyperbaric Oxygen at Different Temperatures *

Chamber Temp.	Chamber Pressure	Mortality %	Convulsed	Convulsion Time	Skin Temp. /6 Hr	Core Temp /6 Hr	Lung Pathology*
8°C	6 ATA	--	84.6%	20.5 ± 4.3	--	--	3+
8°C	3 ATA	--	--	--	-12°C	-11°C	--
8°C	1 ATA	--	--	--	-3°C	-2°C	--
25°C	6 ATA	--	92%	25 ± 6.4	--	--	4+
25°C	3 ATA	17	--	--	-1.5°C	-2°C	2+
25°C	1 ATA	--	--	--	-1°C	-1°C	--
37°C	6 ATA	10	70%	19.3 ± 3.5°	--	--	4+
37°C	3 ATA	83	--	--	+3°CXX	+7°C	1+
37°C	1 ATA	--	--	--	--	--	--

Table 2. Interstitial cuff size of pulmonary vessels following exposure to 6 ATA oxygen

	Vessel lumen size (mm)					
	<20		20-50		50-80	
Vessel type	Artery	Vein	Artery	Vein	Artery	Vein
Cuff thickness+ (mm)	38±4	N.D.*	41±3	18±4	74±5	32±4
Ration of cuff thickness to vessem lumen radius	5.11	--	2.59	1.00	2.35	0.99

+Mean ± SEM
*N.D. = Not detectable

REFERENCES

1. Clark, J.M. (1982). Oxygen Toxicity. In The Physiology and Medicine of Diving. Edited by Bennett, P.B. and Elliott, D.H., p. 200 - 238. Best Publishing Co., San Pedro, CA.
2. Donald, K.W. (1947). Oxygen poisoning in man. I and II. Br. Med. J. 1:667-672; 712-717.
3. Haugaard, N. (1968). Cellular mechanism of oxygen toxicity. Physiol. Rev. 48: 311-373.
4. Clark, J.M. and Lambertsen, C.J. (1971). Pulmonary oxygen toxicity: a review. Pharm. Rev. 23: 37-133.
5. Deneke, S.M. and Fanburg, B.L. (1980). Normobaric oxygen toxicity of the lung. New Eng. J. Med. 303: 76-86.
6. Frank, L. and Massaro, D. (1980). Oxygen toxicity. Am. J. Med. 69: 117-126.
7. Grossman, M.S. and Penrod, K.E. (1949). Relationship of hypothermia to high oxygen poisoning. Am. J. Physiol. 156: 177-181.
8. Kovatchich, G.B. (1980). Depression of 14/CO2 production from [U -14/ C] glucose in brain slices under high pressure oxygen: relationship between metabolic rate and tissue sensitivity to oxygen. J. Neurochem. 34: 459-462.
9. Puglia, C.D., Glauser, E.M. and Glauser, S.C. (1974). Core temperature response of rats during exposure to oxygen at high pressure. J. Appl. Physiol. 36: 149-153.
10. Bailey, C.T., Ordy, J.M. and Haymaker, W. (1975). The effects of cosmic radiation on pocket mice to oxygen and heat. Part IV observations on the brain. Aviat. Space and Environ. Med. 46: 527-528.
11. Harrison, G.A., Corbett, R.L. and Klein, G. (1975). The effects of cosmic particla radiation of pocket mice aboard XVIII. Preflight studies on tolerance of pocket mice to oxygen ahd heat. Part III. Effects on lungs. Aviat. Space and Environ. Med. 46: 520-524.
12. Pinkerton, K.E., Mercer, R.R. and Bennett, P.B. (1986). The pathobiology of hyperbaric oxygen - effects of temperature on sensitivity. Proceedings 9th Symposium of Underwater Physiology, Kobe, Japan. Undersea Medical Society, Bethesda.
13. Theodore, J. and Robin E.D. (1976). Speculation on pulmonary edema (NPE). Am. Rev. Res. Dis. 113: 405-411.

New developments in Hyperbaric Chambers

Dr. Ing. W. Lubitzsch

NEW DEVELOPMENTS IN HYPERBARIC CHAMBERS

Already back in 1913 Drägerwerk started the development of hyperbaric systems with the design and installation of a simulator for 200 m on its own premises for manned equipment tests (Fig. 1).

Here on July 17th, 1917, Dräger Engineers were carried out the first air dive to 79 m with the head of the Engineering Department as one of the test persons. It was the intention to gain more own physiological basic Know How for themselves how pressure effects the human being. Qualified physiological, medical assistance was not available at that time. The original protocol (Fig. 3) of this dive reports about effects of Nitrogen narcosis as well as bends coming and going and about "sleeping legs up the hips" etc. The decompression time was 9 hours after a stop of 10 minutes in 79 m.

Today, research and development regarding hyperbaric systems is carried out in closest cooperation of physiologists, physicians, operators and manufacturers. This guarantees an optimum result for

- standard systems such as the one person treatment chamber (Fig. 4)

or

- the custom made complexes as TITAN (Fig. 5) for medical and physiological research installed in Cologne

or

- GUSI (Fig. 6). In GUSI manned dives successfully were carried out in depths to 600 m last year. It is one of the world's most modern and largest underwater facility.

As a further aspect has to be mentioned new legislation regarding medical equipment in different countries.

On January 1st, 1986, a new legislation governing medical equipment and its application came into force in the Federal Republic of Germany. It states that chamber-systems for HBO are subject to very stringent safety standards as applicable for anaesthesia machines and pacemakers.

This legislation governs especially combinations of different apparatuses in a therapy-system. Only officially approved combinations are allowed.

This is to serve the patient's safety as well as the user's liability interests. The manufacturer, however, is forced to consider and test the effects of the system in the different combinations and conditions. This is all the more important since the need and application of sensitive subsystems for intensive care and monitoring in HBO is growing rapidly.

Basically the development of chambers for HBO has taken two different directions over the past years:
- The walk-in multiplace chamber frequently used for outpatient treatment (Fig. 7) and
- The one person chamber (Fig. 8).

WALK-IN MULTIPLACE CHAMBERS

This chamber type is filled with air, and oxygen respiration is via masks covering the mouth and nose.

An entrance-chamber lock allows patients to enter and leave the main chamber without having to alter the treatment pressure. Medicines, drinks and other items may be passed into the chamber via small air locks.

Modern chamber systems of this type are equipped with comprehensive gas supply and monitoring systems. If a critical component should fail, the patient would not be in danger, since the operator would be able to recognize and rectify the malfunction immediately.

An extensive system of locking and interlocking mechanisms serves to considerably reduce operating errors. Thus all doors close automatically on account of the pressure built-up inside the chamber.

The compressed air supply systems are designed with a double safety feature: So, should the compressor fail, there will be a sufficient supply of compressed air in the high-pressure tanks to finish the chamber session safely.

Particular attention is focused on the danger of fire in the chamber. To begin with, all safety precautions are taken to exclude a potential fire hazard inside the chamber, as it concerns the electricity supply, mechanical friction and electrostatic charging. If an electricity supply is indispensable inside the chamber, the operating voltage is limited to a maximum of 24 V.

Furthermore, only materials which have undergone thorough testing in accordance with specified safety standards are used for blankets and seat coverings etc.

Finally, the immediate elimination with "overboard dump" of the O_2 exhaled by the patients prevents walk-in chambers from becoming enriched with O_2 which in turn would increase the fire hazard. The oxygen content of the chamber air is monitored continuously. A sprinkler system may be provided for the highly unlikely event of a fire occurring despite all built-in safety precautions. In that case masks also act as breathing apparatuses to protect the patients from smoke poisoning.

A good telephone system is not only important from a safety angel but also plays a psychological role. Each individual patient is able to communicate with the outside doctor via headphones without the other patients having to over-hear what the doctor passes on private information. Here again, There is a redundant system in the form of an emergency telephone. If required, light music may be played in via the headphones or instructions can be given as to what to do - in particular with regard to pressure compensation during the compression phase.

The compression rate may be selected as to ensure that none of the patients have to suffer sever earache if they experience difficulties with pressure compensation.

ONE PERSON CHAMBERS

Apart from walk-in chambers, one-man chambers have also become established worldwide, representing the second direction of development. The patient breathes pure oxygen from the chamber without a mask. This type of chamber is being increasingly used to treat severe illnesses and intensive-care patients. The question as to which type of chamber is more suitable for hyperbaric therapy all depends upon local application. Each type of chamber has its own special fields of use, as mentioned above, and hospitals are increasingly using the two systems in parallel.

Despite the confined space inside the chamber, cases of patients suffering a claustrophobia are very rare. A large number of windows permits close visual contact and good speech contact, between the patient and the doctor. The patient also has a good view of everything that is going on in the direct vicinity of the chamber. The doctor, on the other hand, is able to keep the patient under close observation and thus keep himself informed of the patient's condition at all times.

The rate of pressure increase, the treatment pressure and the pressure reduction rates are all implemented automatically on the basis of preset values, so that the doctor in charge is able to devote most of his attention to observing the patients.

The build-up of pressure may be reduced or halted in the event of difficulty with pressure compensation during the initial phase of treatment. The pressure curve is recorded automatically throughout the full duration of treatment.

One-man chambers of the type indicated were developed especially for intensive care and gentle patient handling. A special transport system is used to transport the patient from his bed in the ward to the final treatment position, eliminating repeated patient transfers. If necessary artificial respiration may be conducted during transport and also throughout the full duration of treatment in the chamber. In addition, all other intensive-care key functions may be performed during hyperbaric oxygen treatment.

The system for intensive care respectively monitoring includes units for:
- respiration,
- monitoring of vital data such as EEG, ECG, blood pressure, pulse, breathing rate, respiratory minute volume etc.,
- infusions and transfusions,
- drainage body fluids.

Should the patient require direct intervention on the part of the doctor during treatment, then the chamber pressure can be reduced in a short time without danger of decompression illness, and the chamber opened.

The following points should be noted for purposes of comparing the systems:

Walk-in chambers and their advantages:

*simultaneous treatment of several patients (often outpatients)
*application of treatment which requires the presence of the doctor during therapy (e.g. surgery under high pressure)
*fewer problems with claustrophobia due to the greater space available for treatment

One-man chambers and their advantages:

*they take up less space. Special construction and installation measures of the building are not usually necessary,
*the O_2 supply can generally be taken from the central supply system,
*the outlay on the system, including operating and maintenance costs, is lower,
*fewer operators are required. One, or a maximum of two persons will generally be sufficient,
*decompression procedures do not need to be observed,
*in a one-person chamber the patient is able to breathe freely from the surrounding atmosphere without a mask.

One-person chambers that are filled with O_2 call for greater care in terms of the materials used in order to eliminate any danger of ignition. Here, it is especially important that the chamber operator adheres to materials that have been recommended by the manufacturer.

Now I want to focus on some special subsystems as parts of an integrated therapy system.

A) Ventilators

Ventilation systems are to be regarded as a very special integrated part of HBO-therapy and designed to cope with changing ambient pressure conditions during the therapy. There should be a minimum fluctuation regarding respiration parameters within the normal operating limits.

The Fig. 9 shows as an example the ventilation frequency versus chamber pressure of a standard and modified ventilator (Oxylog resp. Oxylog MOD). As a further parameter the ventilation volume has to be considered.

B) Infusion Pump

The infusion pump is to assure a correct function even when working against a pressure of 3 bars.

C) Blood Pressure Measurement

For non-invasive measurement of the blood pressure Drager developed a unit. A Korotkov-microphone is used under a cuff which can be pressurized from outside.

The systolic and diastolic pressures are to be read when corresponding optic/acoustic signals are given during release of the cuff pressure. The monitoring unit is arranged outside the chamber. The measurement can be carried out completely from outside the chamber.

D) Transcutaneous PO_2 and PO_2 Measurement

$TCPO_2$ measurement which became established for normal clinical use has now also been clinically tested and applied in HBO already in the second generation.

The Drager Oxycapnometer provides two O_2 and one CO_2-sensors to be applied in parallel. The standard-Oxy-capnometer had to be modified regarding O_2 measuring range and the sensor cables which need carefully shielded electrical penetrations. Normally, windows are used for the installation of custom made penetrator flanges.

The clinical tests have proven that valuable information is gained with one O2-sensor (a) attached near the Subclavian artery and the other (b) nearest to the sick part of the body. Sensor a) informs about reading of O2-toxicity limits, sensor b) about the effect of HBO not only during one session but also over a period of several sessions (Fig. 10).

The CO_2-sensor is applied directly near the sensor a) and gives very good and reliable information about the CO_2 during treatment. It is reported that normally the CO_2-pressure in healthy persons is not increased under pressure. However, the CO_2-value increases significantly with bad perfusion or in shock cases. Both ($TCPO_2$ and $TCPOC_2$) values proved very valuable during HBO-treatment (Fig. 2).

Special characteristics compared with the first generation (Oxymeter) are:

-fast response (approx. 15 min.)

-higher stability of the system. No $TCPO_2$-adjustment during one day required,

-applicability of the sensor improved.

End

The duty of manufacturers is considered to develop and offer proven systems for HBO where all subsystems fit to each other in the best possible way. Such a development requires a cooperation of all parties concerned.

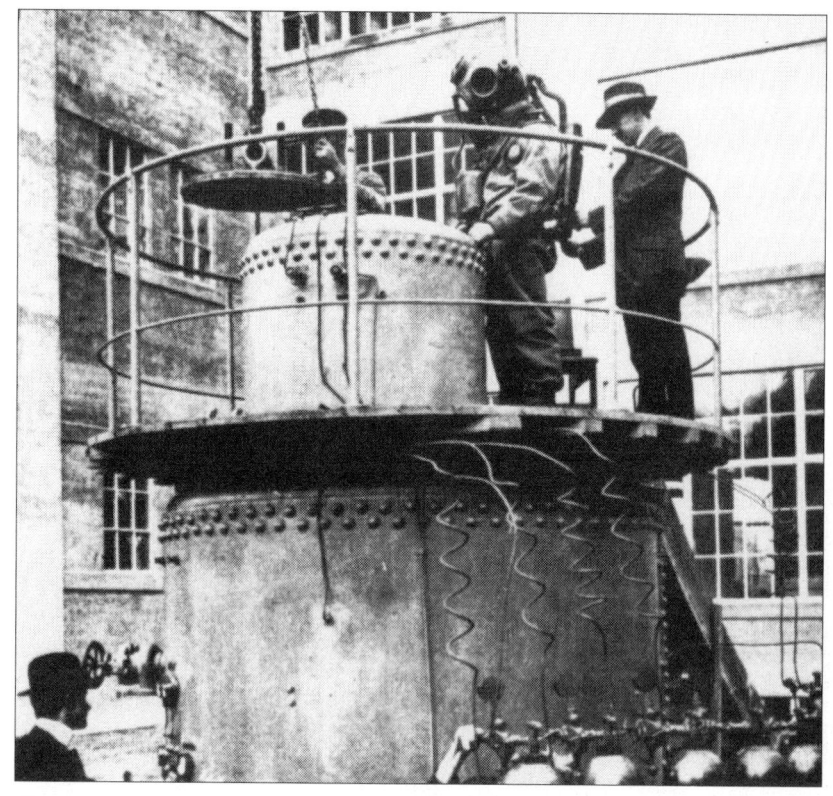

Figure 1 First Draeger Underwater Simulator for 200 m installed 1913

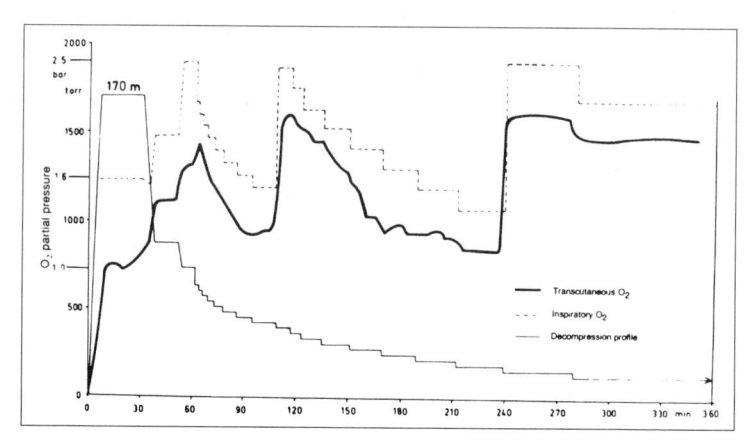

Figure 2 Trend of TcPO$_2$ during a 170 m diver (DFVLR)

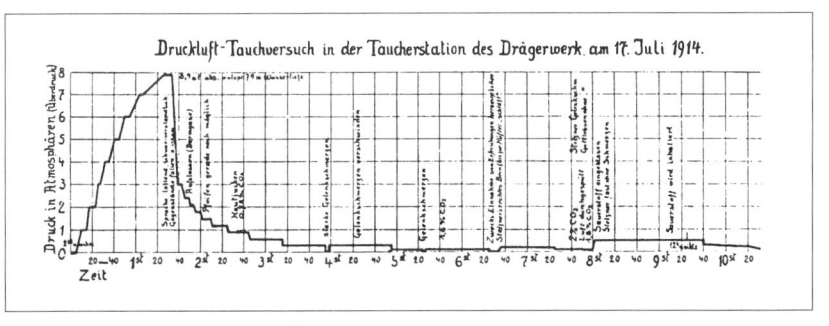

Figure 3 Protocol of a manned dive in 79 m in 1917

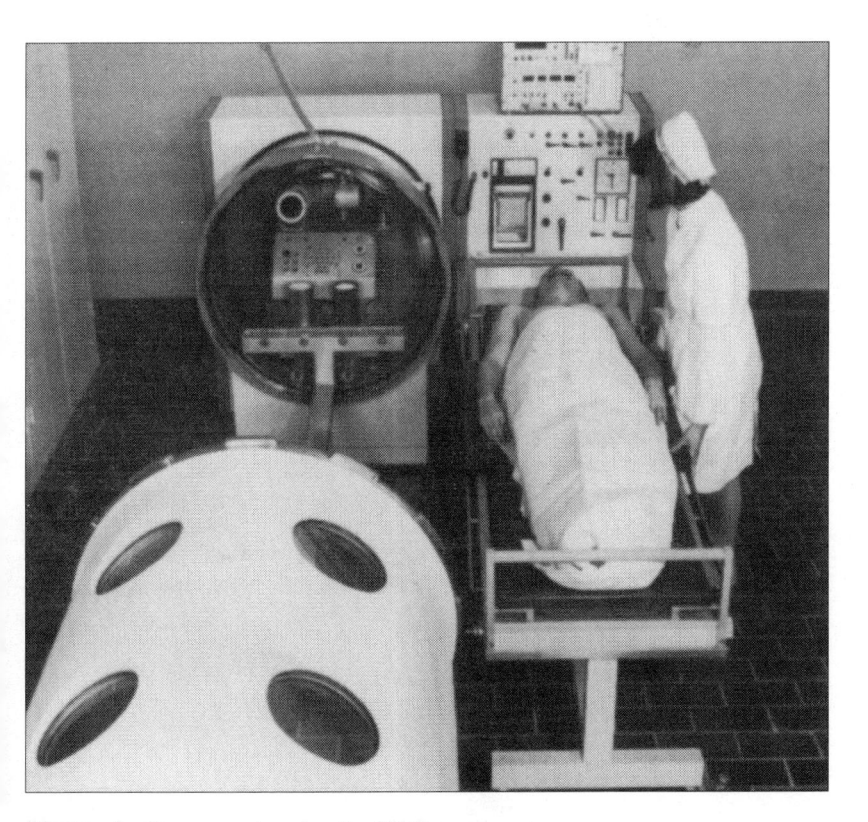

Figure 4 One-man chamber for HBO-treatment

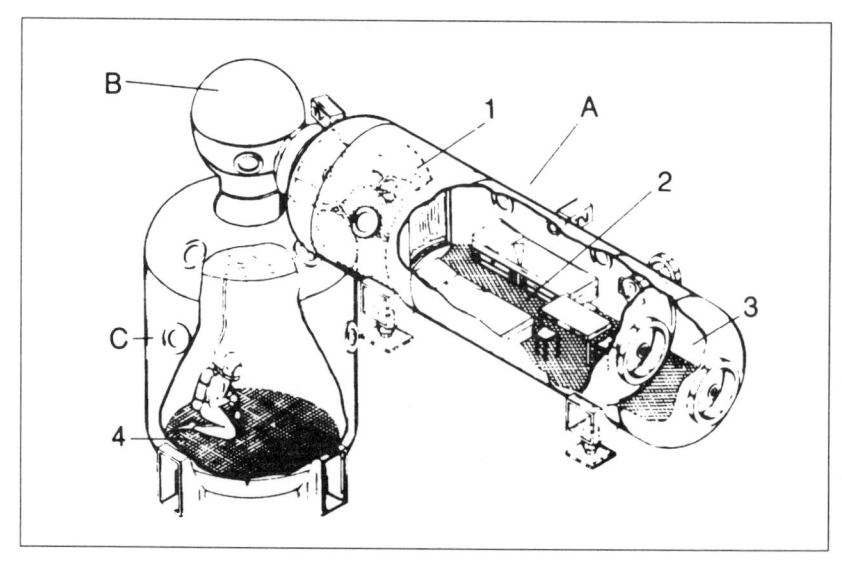

Figure 5 Underwater Simulator TITAN for medical and physiological research

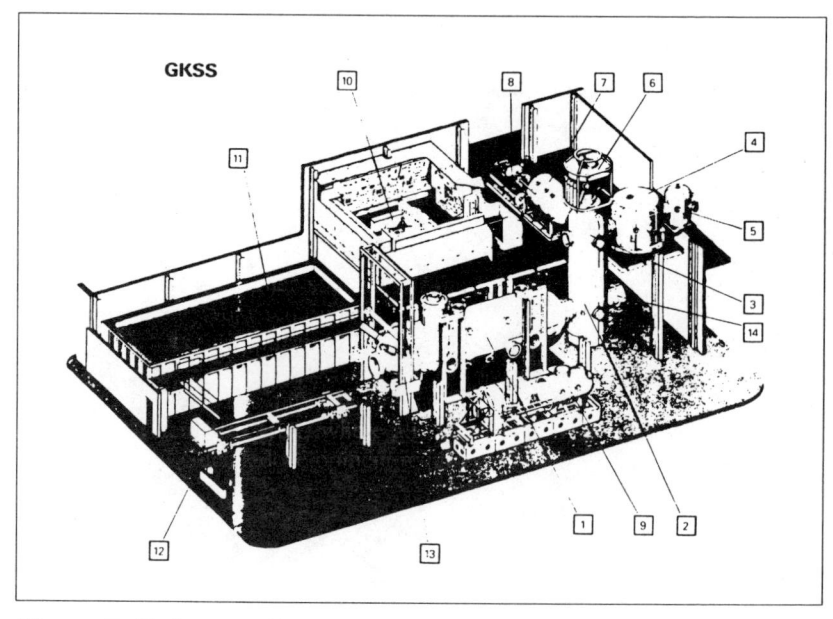

Figure 6 Underwater Simulator GUSI

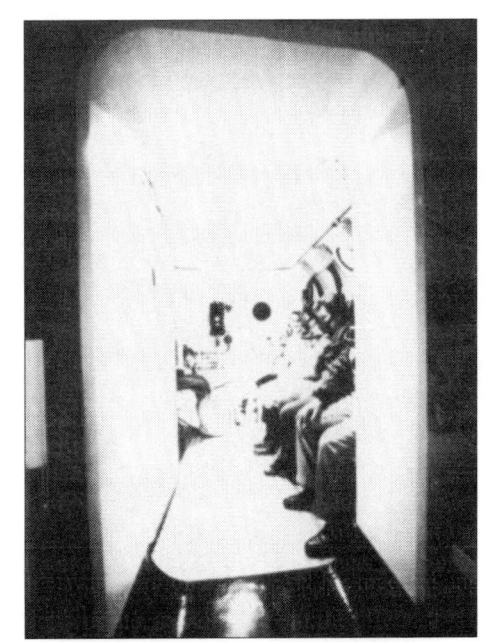

Figure 7 Multiplace chamber

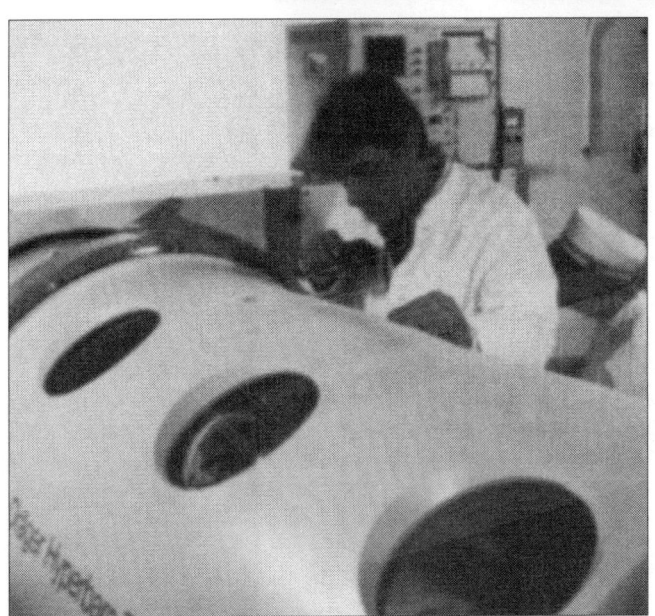

Figure 8 One-man chamber

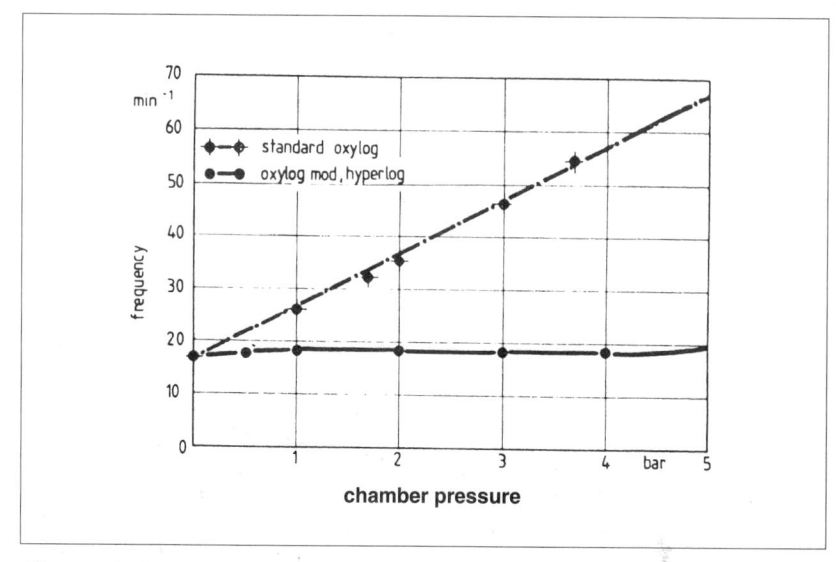

Figure 9 Ventilation frequency versus chamber pressure of the Oxilog resp. Oxilog MOD

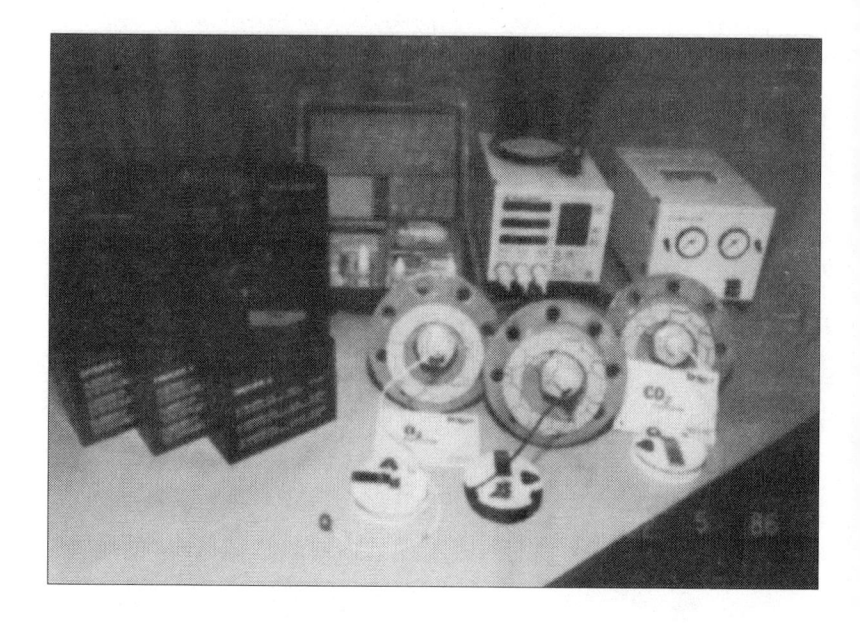

Figure 10 Oxycapnometer set with penetration flanges

# The study of gas leakage test for saturation diving system with air instead of helium

Chen Hong-jun, Yu Hai-Quan, Cui Hai-Liang,
Ren Xiao-Ling and Zheng Ru-Gen
Supervisor: Ni Guo-Tan

Department of Naval Medicine, Second Military
Medical University, Shanghai, China

Rules for certification of diving system require that gas leakage tests have to be carried out with the gas mixture which the system is supposed to contain, and be conducted at the maximum allowable working pressure, that is to say, the mixture contained approximately 95% helium to be used for deep diving system. In this way, it is very expensive.

It is believed that helium leakage can be calculated by multiplying air leakage and 2.65 (according to Graham law, diffusion rate of helium is 2.65 times as fast as that of nitrogen). And some commercial diving organizations suggest that leakage tests be carried out with a mixture containing 10-20% helium instead of mixture containing high concentration helium.

The purpose of this study was to test and verify whether the above mentioned opinions tally with the actual situation and to find cheap gas instead of expensive helium for leakage tests.

METHODS AND RESULTS

The present study has been carried out within 3 compression chambers with different structure at 50-15 kgf/cm^2 with air and 27 kinds of mixture containing various concentrations helium.

1. Chamber A test

The volume of chamber A is 54L. There is a single out-open door and the chamber body and the door are connected by bolts. The leakage gap can be adjusted by bolts. Results here were go under the same leakage gap.

Table 1. Chamber A Test 1, test pressure 25kgf/cm^2

No.	Air or He%** pre-leakage	post-leakage	leakage rate (pressure drop%/4h)	He*leakage/ Air leakage
1 14	Air		1.96 1.77 } $\bar{X}$:1.865	
2	9.60		3.13	1.68
3	81.5		2.75	1.47
4	65.0	64.8	2.46	1.32
5	51.9	51.6	2.38	1.28
6	41.0	41.3	2.19	1.17
7	33.7	34.0	2.24	1.20
8	27.5	27.7	2.21	1.18
9	22.0	21.9	2.21	1.18
10	18.0	18.2	2.20	1.18
11	12.5	12.5	2.16	1.16
12	8.4	8.4	2.02	1.08
13	5.8	5.8	2.01	1.08

* Various concentration helium (the same below)
** The first and the last are air and the rest are helium. In order to observe the change of helium concentration, helium concentration was analyzed by chromatography in pre- and post-test when helium was used (the same below)

Table 2. Chamber A Test 2, test pressure 25kgf/cm^2

No.	Air or He% pre-leakage	post-leakage	leakage rate (pressure drop%/4h)	He leakage/ Air leakage
1 8	Air		1.59 1.54 } $\bar{X}$:1.565	
2	94.8		2.62	1.67
3	58.5	58.5	1.95	1.25
4	35.0	35.0	1.91	1.22
5	20.75	20.75	1.86	1.19
6	12.65	12.65	1.88	1.20
7	8.0	8.0	1.83	1.17

Table 3. Chamber A Test 3, test pressure 25kgf/cm²

	Air or He%		leakage rate	He leakage/
No.	pre-leakage	post-leakage	(pressure drop%/11h)	Air leakage
1	Air		4.08 ⎫ X̄:4.015	
11			3.95 ⎭	
2	95.0		6.64	1.65
3	77.4		5.49	1.37
4	59.0		4.85	1.21
5	40.1	40.1	4.70	1.17
6	30.5		4.62	1.15
7	20.0	20.0	4.18*	
8	16.08	16.03	4.33	1.08
9	12.05	12.03	4.18	1.04
10	8.0	8.0	4.22	1.05

*blunder

Table 4. Chamber A Test 4 25kgf/cm²

	pressure (kgf/cm²)	chamber temperature (degrees C)	He% (in the chamber)
initiation	25.08	14.0	35.7
post 72h	18.57	12.26	35.7

2. Chamber B test

The volume of chamber B is 340L. There is a single inner-open door. The results are shown in table 5.

Table 5. Chamber B Test

	leakage rate (pressure drop%/12h)		
pressure (kgf/cm²)	Air	95%He	He leakage/ Air leakage
50	4.135 ⎫ X̄:4.098	7.266 ⎫ X̄:7.322	
50	4.061 ⎭	7.377 ⎭	1.787
25	2.549 ⎫ X̄:2.633	4.482 ⎫ X̄:4.479	
25	2.717 ⎭	4.476 ⎭	1.701

3. Chamber C test

The volume of chamber C is 7800L (7.8m3). There are two inner-open doors. To save the helium, crammer was used to occupy 4336L of chamber volume and the net volume is only 3464L. The results are shown in table 6.

Table 6. Chamber C Test (net volume, 3464L)

pressure (kgf/cm^2)	leakage rate (pressure drop %/4h) Air	96% He	He leakage/ Air leakage
25	1.129	1.868	1.65
15	0.809	1.336	1.65

Discussion

    1. The results show that the leakage rate of mixture containing helium is higher than that of air under the same conditions. Nine times of test results indicate that 95%-helium-leakage/air-leakage is between 1.65-1.78 is three chambers under the 15-50 kgf/cm^2 condition. It appears that leakage rate can't be calculated by multiplying air leakage rate and 2.65.

    2. Under the same condition, the higher the concentration of helium, the higher the leakage rate is. That helium concentration in the chamber in constant in pre-and post-test suggests that mixtures leak from diving system in original concentration. So we think that the leakage rate of low concentration helium can't directly replace that of high concentration helium.

    3. The regression of chamber A test 1 shows that the specific value (Y) between the leakage rate of mixtures contained various concentration helium and air correlates well (r=O.9447, p<0.01) with helium concentration (x) in the mixtures and Y=10 -1.0249+0.0089 +1 (S=0.034) in 25 kgf/cm^2 condition. We have checked chamber A test 2 and 3 and the maximum absolute error between the theoretical value and the actual value is less than 0.11. It indicates that the formula is very reliable and practical.

    4. When helium concentration is 95%, Y=1.70. It is very close to actual mean value, 1.675 (± 0.023 SD) which is got from 6 test data in three chambers. We suggest that gas leakage test for heliox saturation rate of mixture contained 95% helium be calculated (leakage rate of air times 1.73 (or Y+2S).

    5. The results also indicate that helium-leakage/air-leakage in different leakage gap is very close (1.65-1.70) and it suggests that helium-leakage/air-leakage doesn't correlate with leakage gap volume.

    6. Under different pressure, whether there is certain difference in helium-leakage/air-leakage is further to be tested and verified.

Air transportable emergency hyperbaric treatment systems

Recent Australian experience

I. Millar

National Safety Council
Traralgon, Victoria
Australia

Air Transportable Emergency Hyperbaric treatment systems have often been proposed as a means of reducing delay in providing treatment to those requiring urgent hyperbaric oxygen therapy. A number of these systems have been established, in some cases at great expense, in various parts of the world. For such systems to provide a service which fulfills the goals set, which must primarily include improving patient care without excessive risk, many requirements must be met. Adequate transportable hyperbaric chambers are only one of these. Suitable aircraft, chamber operating and medical teams and their equipment must be available at short notice to respond rapidly to the areas where patients are located. If transfer under pressure (TUP) to larger chambers is part of plan, compatible mating flanges must be available, as must the logistics for effecting TUP. Finally good communications and co-ordination must control the response.

As those who have been involved in such operations know, bringing these factors together and making them work is not easy, and as a result, relatively few transportable chamber systems have been established, and many that have, have seen little use.

Over the last 4 years, 45 patients have been treated and transported in the Eastern Australian region, and I will now describe some of our methods and experience.

Australia is a large country, and recreational SCUBA diving is extremely popular. This, with the abalone diving industry, has generated most of the 150-200 diving-related cases treated in Australian chambers per year. Relatively few static chambers, and the referral of an increasing number of CO poisoning and other urgent cases have created the need for efficient retrieval systems.

The cases described have been handled by the one organization, the National Safety Council of Australia Emergency Services Group (NSCA).

This non-government, non-profit organization supplies a wide range of emergency services to appropriate Australian and oversea authorities. These include airborne fire fighting, search and rescue, remote sensing, medevac and hyperbaric services, and as such, the organization has considerable logistic resources and experience, especially in remote are operations and rapid mobilization.

Bases with hyperbaric retrieval chambers are currently located in Townsville, Wollongong, Sale and Adelaide.

Major static facilities capable of TUP exist at the Australian Institute of Marine Science, Townsville, Royal Australian Navy, HMAS Penguin, Sydney, NSCA Victoria and the Royal Adelaide Hospital, Adelaide.

The NATO bayonet system is used with the flange either incorporated into the chamber or fitted via an adaptor. Most retrievals are carried out on behalf of the appropriate State Ambulance Service, coordinated as necessary by the receiving static hyperbaric unit, or the national Diving Emergency Services (DES). NSCA supply aircraft, two man chambers, operators, and in-chamber attendants who are on base from 7 A.M. till 7 P.M. every day and available on call after hours. In most cases a medical officer with hyperbaric training accompanies cases. Response in approximately half an hour by day and an hour at night can usually be achieved.

The helicopters used are twin-engined, instrument flying equipped Bell 212 or 412 aircraft. Especially in bad weather or at night the combination of such aircraft with a portable HBC can enable a safe, higher IFR retrieval to be used rather than a potentially more dangerous low level mercy flight by a smaller helicopter.

Fixed Wing aircraft are Cargo door Beech King Airs. This Twin turbo prop aircraft has proved a versatile machine with long range and 250 knot speed. It is pressurized, has fairly good short rough airstrip landing capabilities and has proved reliable.

Chambers used to date are Drager duocoms. The basic version of these chambers allow a medical attendant to sit at the head of a patient helping with the use of oxygen BIBS, monitoring the patient and administering I.V. therapy. A communications system and a small medical lock are fitted. A fair degree of airway control should be possible if required however all but the smallest patients are confined to lying on their backs.

Although these chambers have been used successfully in many cases, concerns over management of vomiting, oxygen fits, and the more severely ill patient led us to propose more roomy designs, and Drager have since supplied a larger model, which gives the attendant considerably more room in which to work whilst still fitting into the confines of the aircraft in use. In fact, the attendant can transfer from a sitting position to kneeling at the patients head and the patient can be rolled onto and nursed on his or her side if required which is a great advance. We look forward to trialling the Dive Tech chamber which seems to have promise as a further improvement in this field of portable HBC design.

Based on our experience, continual improvements in associated equipment are being made. Provision for alternate gas supplies, and bypass of faulty regulators is made, although no failures have been experienced to date. Adaptors have alternate types of oxygen and air cylinders are carried. Modifications to improve medical care are also made and as can be seen here can some what reduce the increased room in the large chamber. The oxygen BIBS supply has been modified to provide oxygen to manual or automatic resuscitators. Expired gas is scavenged and bled overboard with a system incorporating a reservoir, safety valve and a control valve.

Through hull, differential pressure powered suction is fitted to some chambers and a compact manual sucker is always available. Small pouches and shelves assist in storage and use of medications, airways and the like, and electrophysiological monitoring leads are fitted. A wide range of general ancillary equipment and spares are carried, including comprehensive medical assessment and treatment equipment. Although paramedical and nursing staff usually act as in chamber attendants, the Medical Officer will fill this role if required for the more severe patient. It is important to remember that single lock chambers do not allow change of attendants before TUP i
n many cases.

Aircraft are fitted with extensive radio communication systems and recent trials of airborne telephones promise further improvement and privacy.

Loading and unloading HBC's can be a problem and is a time of potential hazard especially if the chambers are occupied. We prefer to leave the chamber in the aircraft in the field if possible; however manual handling is possible if enough strong people are available. A flat bed truck is a useful aid. At major airports, baggage handling facilities can be adapted and used successfully. NSCA bases use a variety of mechanical aids, and a recently developed scissor lift platform is rapidly proving to be a safe, effective, versatile and preferred method.

Although the HBC's will fit in a standard ambulance, larger vehicles are preferred for transport from airport to hospital. As the static unit, overhead lifting tackles allow the necessary alignment and rotation for TUP.

Using these systems, successful evacuations from as far away as Rabaul and Fiji have been made as well as many involving thousands of kilometers within Australia. Some relatively short evacuations have also been performed to save exposing patients to altitude. As an example, the road from the coast south of Sydney climbs 500 meters en route over the Illawarra escarpment, making air transport preferred, and in some weather conditions low level helicopter flight may not be safe.

Case severity has varied, but includes 3 ventilated cases including a critically ill gas gangrene patient. All treatments to date have had a successful outcome. Some treatments have been carried out on site, however in most cases evacuation during treatment is preferred, as TUP can then be effected in case of complications and for comfort in diving and other longer treatments.

Alternatively, minimal pressurization to prevent exposure to altitude only can be used where TUP facilities do not exist, and cases such as most non-diving cases who can be safely surfaced can complete a treatment en route, as may happen on longer diving evacuations anyway.

The availability of transportable, add on entry locks holds the promise of allowing pre-placement of evacuation chambers closer to at risk locations, say in regional hospitals, whilst still allowing more experienced attendants to lock in, and evacuation under pressure of difficult cases to occur. We look forward to continuing developments in this field.

Is transport of diving casualties under pressure worth it?

Harry F. Oxer, M.A., F.F.A.R.A.C.S.

Consultant Diving & Hyperbaric Medicine
Fremantle Hospital, Western Australia

Reports of diving accidents in Western Australia since 1980 have been collected and analyzed. The delay between incidents and recompression was estimated, distances travelled and methods of transport were established and final outcomes noted.

Western Australia is a huge State with an area of 1 million square miles (2.5 million square kilometers) but with the small population of 1.4 million. One million of these live in and around Perth, the rest are scattered over a large area. Diving often occurs in very remote areas.

A system of transporting the majority of diving accidents in an air transportable emergency hyperbaric treatment system has been proposed.

Because of the size and remoteness of much of Western Australia, and the fact that diving accidents can happen anywhere, it appeared unlikely that such a system would have much application in Western Australia.

For the past nine years, a protocol for the management of diving accident in Western Australia, and their retrieval to a recompression facility, has existed very successfully. This is based on the use of the Ambulance Service provided by the St. John Ambulance Association, and aircraft of the Royal Flying Doctor Service, mostly pressurized, to retrieve distant patients. Several of these aircraft are already stationed in remote areas and would be able to respond far more quickly than a centrally placed chamber.

All diving accident records since 1980 were examined in retrospectively. The majority were decompression sickness, but several cases of arterial gas embolism were among the group. About half of these cases occurred in and around Perth, but of these outside this area, some were distances of up to 3,000 kilometers away. It was common for there to be delayed reporting of cases, sometimes for many days, and in two cases, some two to three weeks.

During the period under examination, almost all cases were recompressed in the Royal Australian Navy Facility on behalf of the civilian authorities. Almost all cases achieved complete clinical remission of all signs and symptoms. The only cases which did not do so, had either received incomplete treatment, or extremely long delays, in two cases, of more than 3 weeks. By contrast, a number of patients not treated until 3 - 8 days following the incident, still recovered completely as far as clinical signs were concerned, though they usually needed 2, 3, or 4 treatments rather than the one required for patients received earlier.

Reports have been received from some post-mortem examinations which suggest that though clinical remission is obtained, damage may still be present. However, the vast majority of cases appear to respond completely to treatment, despite some delays.

The number of cases examined is small, but this retrospective group of 66 patients produced little evidence to suggest that in Western Australia, a hyperbaric retrieval system would offer advantages. The time to retrieve a distant patient to recompression would not be reduced unless a portable chamber and aircraft could be at each dive site - this would be completely impractical. In addition, under the present system, the outcome in the vast majority of cases, appears to be good despite delays which appear to be inherent in such a remote though scattered population.

The provision of a hyperbaric retrieval system in Western Australia would not seem to confer sufficient advantages to justify its cost at this time.

Hyperbaric oxygen treatment for smoke inhalation in an animal model

Stewart, R. J., Yamaguchi, K. T., Knost, P. M.
Noblett, K. L., Haworth, L. I. and O'Hara, V. S.

Veterans Administration Medical Center,
Valley Medical Center and California State Univ.
Fresno, California, USA
University of California, San Francisco-
Central San Joaquin Valley Medical Education Program

ABSTRACT

Smoke inhalation is known to produce profound pulmonary effects in burn victims. Survival rates of 16 to 25 percent are not uncommon in patients sustaining a significant inhalation injury. Hyperbaric oxygen (HBO) treatment has been used in wound healing procedures and has been considered as treatment for carbon monoxide smoke inhalation. This study investigated the effect of HBO in reducing extravascular lung water (EVLW) formation following an inhalation injury.

Anesthetized and intubated, adult white New Zealand rabbits were allowed to breath cooled cotton smoke until carboxyhemoglobin levels reach 60%. Immediately following, lactated ringers solution, at 5% body weight, was intravenously administered over a two hour period. Three study groups were established: A) Control Group (Smoke & Fluids) B) Smoke, fluids and HBO treatment group and C) Smoke with fluids administered while in the HBO chamber group. The HBO treated groups were placed into a 100% oxygen chamber and taken down to 2.5 atm over 45 minutes, kept at depth for 2 hours, and were then depressurized over a 45 minute period. Group B received fluids before being placed into the chamber while group C received fluids while in the HBO chamber. Control animals, group A, were held at normal atmospheric pressure at room air for an equivalent amount of time.

Once treatment was completed animals were terminated and gravemetric analyses of harvested lungs was performed to determine actual extravascular lung water present. Our results indicate a significant reduction of EVLW in both groups B and C when compared to controls)$p<0.05$). Group B reduced EVLW by 36% while group C reduced EVLW by 66%. Our findings suggest the beneficial role HBO treatment in reducing EVLW accumulation in smoke inhalation and fluid resuscitation model.

INTRODUCTION

Of the estimated 2 million people burned in the U.S. each year, a considerable percentage suffer a concomitant inhalation injury. This combination of external burn and pulmonary injury places the victim at a markedly lessened chance for survival despite the recent advances made in burn treatment and early diagnosis of pulmonary injury (1). The cause of death in this group is nearly always due to the consequences of pulmonary edema (2).

METHODS AND MATERIALS

Adult white New Zealand rabbits ranging in weight from 30 kg - 50 kg were anesthetized with an intramuscular injection of xylazine and ketamine. The ears were shaved and catheters inserted: one into the central artery of one ear, and one into a marginal vein of the opposite ear. Animals were intubated to provide a direct pathway for smoke inhalation and to confine the injury to the lungs. Smoke was generated by burning cotton under reduced airflow in a combustion chamber and then transferred to a cooling chamber. From here the smoke was inhaled directly into the animals lungs for two 2 minute intervals with a 1 minute rest between. Following this procedure a blood same was taken for carboxyhemoglobin determination. COHb levels of at least 60% but no more than 70% were obtained thus indicating a significant inhalation injury. A level this high in humans is nearly always fatal. Immediately following smoke inhalation animals received lactated ringer's solution (at 5% body weight) which was intravenously infused over a 2 hour period. Those animals receiving fluid therapy prior to HBO treatment were given the fluids over the 2 hour period before being placed in the chamber for treatment. Those animals receiving fluids while in the HBO chamber were immediately placed into the period while simultaneously receiving HBO treatment. HBO treatment protocol consisted of pressurizing the animal to 2.5 atmospheres over a 45 minute period using pure oxygen. The pressure was held constant for one hour followed by a 45 minute decompression. Control animals were given smoke and fluids and were at room air for an equivalent length of time.

Following HBO treatment, the animals were terminated and the lungs harvested. Gravimetric analyses of the lungs gave extravascular lung water calculated from wet and dry lung weights with correction made for lung versus blood hemoglobin levels. The value is standardized by dividing the extravascular lung water value by the dry lung weight.

RESULTS

Statistics of gravimetric analyses are shown below. The extravascular lung water is significantly reduced in both groups receiving HBO treatment when compared to the control group only receiving smoke and fluids ($p<0.05$). As can be seen, the animal group receiving fluids while in the chamber reduced extravascular lung water to a greater extent than those animals receiving fluids prior to HBO treatment.

DISCUSSION

Pulmonary edema, which is simply the gathering of abnormally large amounts of fluids in the extra vascular spaces of the lungs, is a common consequence in burn victims suffering a severe inhalation injury, and is the leading cause of death of people of this group (2). The fluid in the extravascular spaces of the lungs interferes with normal gas exchange and can further lead to such complications as pneumonia and respiratory failure. Normal treatment of burn patients necessitates the continuous administration of large volumes of fluid to maintain vital signs. However, this type of fluid loading adds an additional insult to the already damaged lung tissue and often results in a worsened pulmonary edema condition in inhalation injured patients.

A thermal pulmonary injury is rare due to the low heat energy of gases and the tremendous heat dissipating ability of the respiratory tract (3). Rather most injuries incurred by fire victims arise from damage to the endothelial cells of the lungs. These cells play a crucial role in the exchange of oxygen and carbon dioxide and when injured, cannot effectively carryout their vital function resulting in reduced gas exchange. The damage of these cells may be caused directly by inhaling the chemical product of the fire itself, or indirectly by chemicals released in our body in response to injury. The type of structural changes described in this type of injury include gap foundation in the endothelial cell layer, swelling and blebbing, disruption and even loss of endothelial cells. This type of damage increases the permeability of fluid into the extravascular spaces of the lungs and is thus appropriately termed high permeability pulmonary edema. This differs from high pressure or cardiogenic pulmonary edema which is common consequence of congestive heart failure.

The inhalation of toxic products from fires causes approximately 80% of the fire fatalities occurring annually in the U.S. (2). It has been estimated that 77% of deaths having combined burns and smoke inhalation should have survived the burn injury (2). Hyperbaric oxygen treatment, normally used for treating carbon monoxide poisoning, has been shown to reduce morbidity in burn patients treated with HBO. Numerous laboratory and clinical studies have also shown HBO treatment to have a beneficial role increasing the healing rate of external tissue damage such as those caused by burns or extravasation of chemotherapeutic agents (4,5). The actual modality by which HBO conveys its effects is unknown, it may be due to the environment of oxygen or decrease in pressure keeping the fluid within the lung's microvessels.

Our laboratory results of animals receiving HBO treatment supported the indications of earlier studies demonstrating a significant reduction in extravascular lung water following an inhalation injury and thus may be an important therapeutic treatment for victims with smoke inhalation injuries.

CONCLUSION

Our laboratory developed an animal model of inhalation injury and subsequent fluid therapy employing HBO treatment to reduce extravascular lung water accumulation. The results of our study demonstrate that HBO treatment significantly reduces extravascular lung water following an inhalation injury. These results suggest the beneficial role HBO may have as a clinical treatment for patients suffering an inhalation injury.

Table 1.

TREATMENT	N	EVLW/DW	% REDUCTION	
Normals Controls	5	1.35	—	
(Smoke & Fluids)	10	2.52	—	
HBO (Smoke & Fluids)	10	2.10*	36	
HBO (Smoke & Fluids in Chamber)	8	1.75	8	66

* $p<0.05$

REFERENCES

1. Achauer, B.M., Allyn, P.A., Furnas, D.W., et al. Pulmonary complications of burns. Ann. Surg. 177:311 (1972).
2. Formosa, P.J., Waxman, K. Inhalation injuries in burn patients. Hosp. Physician July: 69 (1986).
3. Genovesi, M.G., Effects of smoke inhalation. Chest 77:335 (1980).
4. Knighton, D.R., Hunt, T.K., Regulation of would angiogenesis-effect of oxygen gradients and inspired oxygen concentrations. Presented to the society of University Surgeons, Hershey, PA, Feb. 12-14 (1981).
5. Gong C., Yamaguchi, K.T., Nguyen, et al. Effects of hyperbaric oxygen on adriamycin-induced skin lesions in an animal model. J. Hyperbaric Medicine 1:99 (1986).

Carbon monoxide poisoning in New York City treatment with hyperbaric oxygen

E. Converse Pierce, II, M.D. and William H. Bensky, P.A.

From the Department of Surgery
Mount Sinai School of Medicine of the City of University of New York

ABSTRACT

Since 1983 the North American Hyperbaric Center (NAHC) (affiliated adjacent Bronx Municipal Hospital Center (BMHC)) has provided hyperbaric oxygen (HB) for CO patients meeting Emergency Medical System (EMS) criteria (1): 1. Unconscious or CNS derangement (any carboxyhemoglobin level ([COHb])), 2. [COHb] 25% or more, and 3. Pregnant (any [COHb]. Through 1984, 39 CO patients received HBO; in 1985, 81 were treated including 8 pregnant, and 16 pediatric. CO sources were: fire, 43; heater, 21; engine, 17. 42 of 59 acute patients were in coma; 16 required CPR. Time to HBO averaged 5 hrs. Mean hospital [COHb] was 31% for acute, 28% for chronic, 15% for pregnant patients. Mean maximum [COHb] was 51% for acture, 40% for chronic patients. Mean half time value for [COHb] was 2.1 hrs, roughly equivalent to receiving 64% oxygen. HBO was typically 46 min at 3 ATA (two [COHb} half times), presented few problems, and gave rapid clinical improvement. 13 of 19 stuporous or comatose patients were responsive post HBO and [COHb] became 1.8%. Brain damage was noted twice and there were 4 pediatric deaths. Despite unequal access to HBO in different boroughs, frequent delay, and poor follow-up, EMS efforts to make HBO available for CO poisoning is a success.

Before NY EMS initiated emergency CO procedures in 1983 few CO patients received HBO. In 4 years to September 1986, 181 cases were treated. The 81 1985 cases are reported here:

MATERIALS AND METHODS

68 of the 81 cases were referred from 15 hospitals in the 5 Boroughs of NYC (Table 1), generally directly to the NAHC after BMHC consultation (assisted by the NYC Poison Control Center). After HBO, patients were usually admitted to BMHC.

The NAHC patient HBO unit is somewhat Spartan upright cylinder (diameter 9 ft) that accommodates 2 patients on stretchers, or 5 sitting. The basic treatment plan was 2.8 or 3 ATA for two COHb "half lives" or 46 min. Clinical condition was coded from grade 1 to 5 with a numerical score for each grade:

Grade 1: neurological negative, symptoms minor, score 0.
Grade 2: some confusion or abnormal behavior, score 1.
Grade 3: disoriented with memory loss, weakness, or incoordination, but responsive to commands, score 3.
Grade 4: stuporous with limited responsiveness, often combative when intubated, score 5.
Grade 5: comatose, not responsive or to pain only, score 10.

Cases exposed 3 hrs or less were considered acute. Half time CO removal from hemoglobin (tl/2) was calculated when 2 [COHb] values were available. The maximum [COHb] level (Max [COHb] at the scene was determined when data permitted.*

RESULTS

Source of cases and numbers:
BMHC provided 26% of patients. Altogether 41% were from 4 Bronx hospitals, 43% from 11 hospitals in 3 of the 4 other boroughs (Table I), and 12% from 5 hospitals outside NYC.

* Calculations:

Assumptions:
[COHb] decays exponentially
Rate of decay is inversely proportional to the PIO_2 in mm Hg tl/2 for air (approximately 20% O_2) at 1ATA = 5 hours

Equations:

tl/2 = 1n2 x t / (1nCO1 - 1nCO$_2$)   (1)
O_2% administered = 100 / tl/2   (2)
Max [COHb] [COHb] x 2 (T/tl/2)   (3)

Where:

tl/2 = half time decay [COHb] in hours
ln = the natural logarithm
CO1 = the 1st [COHb] in %
CO2 = the 2nd [COHb] in %
t = the time in hours between [COHb] determinations
T = hours from removal to [COHb] determination
[COHb] = hemoglobin combined with CO in %
Max [COHb] = [COHb] = T= O

Source of CO:
43 patients, all acute, were exposed to CO from fires, 21 from heaters (10 chronic), and 17 from engine exhausts (6 chronic). No exposure was definitely suicidal.

Hours exposed:
The duration of exposure was known or could be estimated in 79 instances. It was 3 hours or less in 54; 3 to 10 hours in 8, an done to 6 days in 12. All fire exposures were acute; most of those to central heaters were chronic.

COHb and tl/2 [COHb] determinations:
A timely [COHb] was obtained in 66 (81%) patients. The calculated mean tl/2 for 15 paired [COHb] was 2.1 ± 4.1 hrs, consistent with the administration of 63.5 ± 35.3% O_2.

Severity of poisoning:
The initial condition of the 54 acute victims is shown in Table IIA. 73% were grade 5 and only 4 grade 1 or 2. The mean severity score was high (8.7) as were the [COHb] (31.4%) and the Max [COHb] (50.7%). Initially, only 3 of the 17 chronic exposures were grade 5 while 7 were grades 1 or 2. The mean score was only 3.6 but mean [COHb] (28.0%) and Max [COHb] (40.1%) were surprisingly high.

The pregnant women were only grade 1 or 2 at the site (mean score 0.4 but the [COHb] was 15.3% and the Max [COHb] 23.4%.

Time and transportation data:
The mean time from removal to the start of HBO was 4.5 hrs for acute, 7.3 hrs for chronic (excluding one of 14 days), and 4.9 hrs for pregnant patients. More than 3 hrs was hospital and the rest transportation time (usually EMS ambulance or helicopter) or NAHC delay (mean 22.3 min).

Status of patients on arrival at the chamber:
The clinical condition of selected patient groups at the time of delivery to the chamber is shown in Table II. Of the acute (non-pregnant) patients, only 19 were still grade 5 (mean score 5.4). The mean severity score of the 17 chronic (non-pregnant) patients had fallen from 3.6 to 1.5; none were still grade 5. 29 patients (all acute, mostly grades 4 or 5) were intubated. Some children had had CPR (13 still grade 5). Mean O_2 administration had been for 2.7 hours.

HBO Treatment:
Thirty-seven treatments were for a single patient, 7 for 2 patients, 4 for 3 patients, 2 for 4 patients, and 2 for 5 patients. The average treatment duration was 75 min. Valium and morphine were used to control agitation or pain in intubated patients receiving mechanical ventilation. Occasionally, discomfort from pressure changes made it expedient to remain at 2ATA for 90 min or to reduce the duration of HBO. Barotrauma to the ears occurred occasionally.

Condition and [COHb] after HBO:
13 of the 19 patients grade before 5 HBO were grade 3 or 4 afterwards. Grade 1 and 2 increased from 11 to 23. Mean severity score fell to 3.1. Post-treatments [COHb] averaged 1.8 and was never elevated. All 17 chronic, and 7 of 8 pregnant patients, were grade 1 after the HBO.

Short-term follow-up:
A check was made on 80 patients at 1 to 4 days. There were 4 deaths and 14 surviving patients had significant hospital complications. Two required prolonged intubation, 2 developed asthma, and 43 developed pneumonia. There was evidence of brain damage in 2 patients that survived. 4 deaths occurred in children who had required CPR and had a longer than average delay (7.5 hours).

Special Categories:
Pregnant patients: 5 were acute and 3 chronic exposures. Four were related to fires and there was one respiratory burn. Two cases resulted from faulty central heaters and 2 from engine emissions. All but 3 (grade 2) were initially grade 1. One patient (100 hrs central heater exposure) had a 30% Max [COHb] and was still grade 2 after HBO.

Pediatric age group (Table IIB): 23 of 30 patients, 5 months to 18 years, were acute. Mean Max [COHb] was 46.1%. 21 were grade 5; 11 of these required CPR. Three were burned. Mean severity score was 9.3. This had fallen only to 7.1 before HBO and was still 4.7 afterwards. Four, persistently grade 5, patients died by the fourth post HBO day. 3 others who were post-CPR has prolonged recoveries and one was permanently brain damaged. A higher prognosis was poorer than for adults who had CPR. 18 acute patients, including 6 given CPR, and all 7 chronic exposures, recovered.

Burns (Table IIC): 18 CO patients were also burned. 10 were surface, 7 respiratory, and one combined burns. One respiratory burn victim was pregnant. Initially grade 2, with a [COHb] of 25%, intubation was not needed, and she did well. The 17 others were initially grade 5 (severity score 10), and 4 required CPR. Mean [COHb] was 35% and Max [COHb] 49%. 12 required intubation, several had problems with inspissated secretions and soot during HBO, and one required extubation for tube obstruction. HBO gave a dramatic decrease in severity score to 3.2 and there were none still grade 5. IV fluids were given without interruption and there was no evidence of dehydration or shock in any of these patients. Two developed pneumonia and one later had asthma. Otherwise, all were improved at 3 or 4 days.

DISCUSSION

There are hidden dangers in CO poisoning, to the CNS (2-4) and to the fetus (5). Oxygen is the established therapy (6,7). Haldane in 1895 (8), on the basis of convincing animal experimentation, stated: "The poisonous action of carbonic oxide (CO) diminishes as the oxygen tension increases, and vice versa." The data reported here serve to emphasize the more rapid therapeutic action of HBO. The average tl/2 for hospital "100%" O_2 was 2.1 hrs (SD 4.0), equivalent to 63.5 ± 35.3% OW2Q. [COHb] fell from 30.6 to 16.8% in 1.5 hrs. The mean severity score fell 63% in 4.5 hrs pre-HBO and 43% in 1.3 hrs of HBO. The post-HBO [COHb] averaged only 1.9%.

Referral of cases meeting the EMS criteria for HBO was incomplete (Table I). The relationship between CO deaths and HBO treated cases varied greatly in different boroughs. For example, 48.5% of NYC HBO cases were from the Bronx which had only 15.8% of the deaths. If the ratio of treated cases had been uniformly as high as in the Bronx, 216 CO patients would have received HBO.

We have only achieved a very short term post-HBO observation of CO patients. This is a major deficiency that needs to be corrected. Nevertheless, an overall assessment of the EMS HBO program is that it has been very effective for the CO cases referred. Emergency HBO in NYC has been successfully inaugurated.

CO Poisoning in New York City

Table 1. New York City HBO treatments for CO in 1985 vs deaths from CO and smoke inhalation 1981-49

	CO Patients Treated HBO		1981-4 Deaths CO & Smoke Inhalation	
BRONX	33	(48.5%)	74	(15.8%)
BROOKLYN	12	(17.6%)	186	(59.8%)
MANHATTAN	16	(23.5%)	79	(16.9%)
QUEENS	7	(10.3%)	111	(23.8%)
STATEN ISLAND	0	-	17	(3.6%)
Total	68	100%	467	100%

CO Poisoning in New York City

Table 2. Clinical grade & mean severity score of CO patients (pregnant women excluded)

GRADE	AT SITE	AT CHAMBER	AFTER HBO
A. 54 ACUTE CASES			
1	2	4	13
2	2	7	10
3	4	12	13
4	1	12	12
5	45	19	6
SEVERITY SCORE	8.7	5.4	3.1

B. 23 ACUTE PEDIATRIC CASES

1	0	0	1
2	1	2	5
3	1	4	4
4	0	4	8
5	21	13	5
SEVERITY SCORE	9.3	7.1	4.7

C. 17 PATIENTS WITH BURNS

1	0	0	1
2	0	0	2
3	0	5	9
4	0	6	5
5	17	6	0
SEVERITY SCORE	10	6.2	3.2

BIBLIOGRAPHY

1. Emergency Medical System City of New York. EMS Advisory No. 5. July, 1984.*
2. Pierce, E.C. II Notes on carbon monoxide (CO) poisoning, especially the importance of early vigorous therapy. Emergency Medical System City of New York. Hyperbaric Advisory Committee Report. May 10, 1985.
3. Smith, J.S. and Brandon, S. Morbidity from acute carbon monoxide poisoning at three-year follow-up. Brit Med J, 1: 318-321, 1973.
4. Lacey, D.J. Neurological sequelae of acute carbon monoxide intoxication. Am J Dis Child, 135, 145-47, 1981.
5. Longon, L.D. The biological effects of carbon monoxide poisoning on the pregnant woman, fetus, and newborn infant. Am J Obstet Gynecol, 129: 69-103, 1977.
6. Behnke, A.R. and Saltzman, H.A. Hyperbaric oxygenation (concluded). New Engl. J Med, 276: 1478-84, 1967.
7. Hyperbaric Oxygen Therapy. A committee report. Chairman: R.A.H. Myers, Undersea Medical Society, Inc. Bethesda, Md. Revised 1986.
8. Haldane, J. The relation of the action of carbonic oxide to oxygen tension. J. Physiol, 18: 201-17, 1895.
9. Deaths due to carbon monoxide and smoke, New York City, 1981-84. Communication from Lee, J.C., NYC Dept. Health (125 Worth St., NYC 10013) to Hyperbaric Center Advisory Committee (NYC EMS). From NYC Dept. Health database.

*Available from EMS, 911 Evaluation Unit, Bellevue Hospital, New York, NY 10016.

Cerebral thrombosis treated by hyperbaric oxygenation

Wen-Ren Li, M.D.

A Report of 490 Cases
Fujian Provincial Hospital
Fuzhou, China

Cerebral thrombosis is a common obstructive cerebral vascular disease which recovers very slowly and usually results in some degree of disability. It is reported that Hyperbaric Oxygenation therapy has a definite beneficial effect on the disease. From February 1980 to June 1986 we treated 490 patients by HBO with gratifying results.

CLINICAL MATERIALS:

The diagnosis of all 490 patients was confirmed by a neurologist. There were 390 male and 100 female patients with ages varying from 28-79 years. As to the duration of the disease, 177 cases were within one month, 65 within 1-2 months, 82 within 3-6 months, 48 within 6-12 months, 37 within 1-3 years and 32 were over 3 years. The symptoms and signs were disturbance of consciousness and mentality, asphasia, etc. In 65% of the patients myodynamia reached 3 degrees while the rest were below 3 degrees. Diagnosis was made by the typical clinical symptoms and signs, and was confirmed by the neurologists. Some patients were examined by CT scanning.

METHOD OF TREATMENT:

Patients were treated with Hyperbaric Oxygenation at 2.5 ATA for 90 minutes with a break of 15 minutes in between daily. One therapeutic course consisted of 15 treatments. The patients usually took 3-4 courses of treatment and rarely any more.

EVALUATION OF THERAPEUTIC EFFECT:

Completely cured.
The symptoms and signs disappeared completely. Patients lead normal, active lives without difficulties.

Markedly improved.
Most of the symptoms and signs disappeared. Myodynamia improved more than 2 degrees.

Improved.
>The symptoms and signs disappeared partially. There was some difficulty in walking. The patient could not entirely care for himself. Myodynamia improved less than 2 degrees.

No effect.
>There was no improvement in the symptoms and signs.

RESULTS:

There were 108 patients completely cured (22%), 157 markedly improved (32%), 166 improved (33.9%), and 59 had no effect (12.1%). The total effective rate was 88%. We compared the effect of HBO therapy and conventional treatment with conventional treatment alone in 50 cases. In a group of 25 cases who received HBO and conventional treatment, 10 patients markedly improved and 15 improved. In the other group of 25, who received conventional treatment alone however, only four patients showed marked improvement, 19 improved and two showed no effect at all. It is evident that HBO with conventional treatment achieves a better effect than conventional therapy alone.

DISCUSSION:

Cerebral artery thrombosis is a common disease affecting people 40 years and over, usually resulting in some degree of disability. Hyperbaric Oxygenation treatment is generally beneficial to these patients by increasing oxygen tension, content and permeability of blood oxygen, thus improving the hypoxic or anoxic state of the cells of the various organs including the brain tissue, and facilitates repair of damage brain tissue. Results of this study showed that the effective rate of HBO therapy is 88%. The response of HBO therapy is related to the duration of the disease. The shorter the duration the better the HBO result. Patients showed very good response when the disease duration was within three months, although this does not mean that patients with longer illness duration do not respond to HBO therapy. The patient whose illness was longer than eight years achieved marked improvement after five courses of HBO therapy. The criteria for selecting patients for HBO treatment should not be too rigid. The response of HBO therapy is closely related to the number of treatments. Most patients respond immediately after the first course, always achieving noticeable improvement after the second and third therapeutic courses. Though there were responses to treatment after the third course, the effects were not as marked as those of shorter duration.

Does hyperbaric oxygen therapy prevent carbon monoxide brain injury?

Cohn, Gerald H., M.D.
Director of Clinical Hyperbaric
Research and Senior Consultant
Geisinger Medical Centre
Danville, Pennsylvania 17822

Cera, Peter J., M.D.
Assistant Chairman of the
Department of Laboratory Medicine
Geisinger Medical Centre
Danville, Pennsylvania 17822

Ehler, William, DVM
Chief of Surgical Research and
Veterinary Hyperbaric Medicine
Clinical Investigation Facility
Wilford Hall
U.S. Air Force Medical Centre
Lackland Air Force Base, Texas

Hubbard, Eugene B., DVM, LTC, VC
Chief of Comparative Medicine Branch
U.S. Army Institute of Surgical Research
Fort Sam Houston, Texas

Shiumazu, Takeshi, M.D.
Research Investigator at U.S. Army
Institute of Surgical Research
Fort Sam Houston, Texas

Storts, R.W., DVM, Ph.D.
Professor of Pathology, Neurophathology
Department of Pathology
College of Veterinary Medicine
College Station, Texas

Widden, S.J., M.D., Ph.D.
Senior Researcher
JESM, Baro Medical Research Institute
New Orleans, Louisiana

Touhey, J.E., Col.
U.S. Air Force M.C.
Chief of Hyperbaric Medicine Division
U.S. Air Force School of Aerospace
Medicine
Brooks Air Force Base, Texas

DOES HYPERBARIC OXYGEN TREATMENT PREVENT OR MODIFY BRAIN INJURY IN CARBON MONOXIDE POISONING?

It has been well established, from both animal (1-3) and clinical studies (4-12) that carbon monoxide produces injury to the central nervous system and that certain areas of the brain are more predisposed to injury than others (1).

THE PREDISPOSED AREAS OF INJURY INCLUDE: (1,2,5)

1. Periventricular white matter lesions.
2. Cellular changes in the basal ganglia including the globus pallidus, substantia nigra, and the red nucleus.

3. Cellular changes in Sommer's sector of Ammon's horn of the temporal lobe.
4. Cerebral edema with terminal herniation from increased pressure.

We are led to believe from these clinical studies that hyperbaric oxygen therapy prevents carbon monoxide encephalopathy (8-11). In an attempt to study this premise in a controlled animal model (HBO2 prevents CO encephalopathy) we have started our studies as follows:

1. Developing an animal model, with consistent reproducibility.
2. Defined protocols similar to our clinical cases which present to our hyperbaric chambers for treatment of carbon monoxide poisoning.

METHODOLOGY

1. Use of adult sheep - (a) anesthetized, (b) intubated, (c) ventilated.
2. Poisoned with pure gas mixture of 500 ppm carbon monoxide and air for selected periods of time - (a) short 5 minute duration, (b) 5 hours, (c) 10 hours.
3. Following poisoning, ventilated on air for three more hours.
4. Animal sacrified with KCL injected into central venous line.
5. Physiological monitoring - (a) carboxyhemoglobin immediately after poisoning (peak level) and repeated at end of three hours' ventilation on air, (b) blood gases and pH, (c) pulmonary arterial pressure, (d) cardiac output, (e) arterial pressures, (f) animal autopsied, (g) heart and lungs studies, (h) brain fixed and stained with 15 selected areas of study.

FINDINGS TO DATE (TOTAL OF EIGHT ANIMALS)

1. Short-term exposures — less than 5 minutes (500 ppm) — no discernible lesions. (4)
2. 500 ppm, 5 hours — early changes in the Purkinje's cells, slight increase in eosinophilia of the cytoplasm. (2)
3. 10 hours (500 ppm) — definite loss of Purkinje's cells, marked changes in the cytoplasm and nucleus of these cells. (2)

COMMENTS OF METHODOLOGY

The animal model and methodology designed shows definite end point injuries to the brain which can be quantitated and localized. We have developed this animal model with reproducible lesions that can be predicted, measured, and hopefully show the "if and how" of hyperbaric oxygen modification of brain lesions.

In this first part of our long-term studies, we have described our animal model and report our preliminary findings; the results are inconclusive and naturally raise many questions.

These successful preliminary findings show that our animal model is reproducible, predictable, and can be correlated quantitatively and qualitatively with dose and time of carbon monoxide poisoning. While monitoring several parameters of shock and tissue oxygenation which are thought to be associated with the underlying pathological processes, our methodology allows us to study prolonged high-dose exposure to the poison with survival of the animal and finding definite measurable neuropathological lesions.

DISCUSSION

NEUROPATHOPHYSIOLOGY

From the review of the literature and our studies to date, which are limited in numbers, we suggest that there are two major types of neuropathology secondary to carbon monoxide poisoning.

TYPE 1 — ACUTE LARGE DOSE POISONING (MAY BE LETHAL)

This poisoning, similar to the cases that are seen in a fire which is so sever that the CO overwhelms the patient and the cytochrome oxidase system is affected in all of the body cells including the brain.

There is anoxia which develops especially in the tissues with a high metabolic rate — i.e., heart and brain. This tissue anoxia affects all of the tissues of the body and as oxygen is restored to the body, certain tissues will return in function but others will not. Certain tissues are more susceptible to this irreversible change, mainly the heart and the brain.

When these large dose poisoning animals are resuscitated the heart, kidneys, and other organs regain function, but the brain may or may not regain function. There may be both neuronal and glial injury. After all tissues are finally rid of the CO, the brain has sustained a cellular injury, to such an extent, it does not return to function. No matter how well the tissues of the body are perfused and have returned to function, the brain, being more sensitive sustains injury during this low-perfusion-hypoxic state of shock at the cellular level and causes delayed demyelination.

Our conjecture as to the underlying pathophysiology is that myelin has an oxygen dependent system, i.e., the "cement" substance that holds the myelin sheath is an ATPase oxygen dependent system, and that injury to the ATPase system is what causes the delayed demyelination seen in the CO poisoning and the periventricular leukomalacia seen in carbon monoxide poisoning.

TYPE II — LOW DOSE; REPETITIVE CHRONIC SOAK (DEBILITATING BUT USUALLY NOT IMMEDIATELY LETHAL)

The second type of neuropathology which we propose is repetitive intermittent low-dose CO poisoning, i.e. the traffic policeman, a leaking furnace exhaust, or a leaking automobile exhaust. Here, there is a repetitive low-dose, but accumulative poisoning, we call the "chronic-repetitive-long term soak." In these cases there is selective neuronal damage where neurons in certain parts of the brain seem to be involved more than others, i.e. basal ganglia, caudate and putamen, substantia nigra, red nucleus, Sommer's sector of Ammon's horn, and the Purkinje's cells of the cerebellum.

Type 1 poisoning (high-dose acute) seems to be related to lack of perfusion, shock, acute anoxia, resulting in total body tissue poisoning, i.e., poisoning of all tissues including the brain.

Type II low-dose, repetitive "long soak," is associated with a more selective poisoning. Certain areas of the brain seem to be more susceptible than others.

We plan to evaluate the role of hyperbaric oxygen treatment in both types of cases and see how it might modify the associated pathology.

Questions Raised So Far From These Preliminary Findings Are:
1. What are the direct effects and the pathophysiological role of carbon monoxide on the brain?
2. Is the resultant pathology from a direct effect of CO, anoxia, shock, hypoperfusion, or a combination of all these factors?
3. Is the pathology related to shock, alterations of the blood brain barrier, or cerebral edema?
4. Does the HBO treatment modify or prevent it?
5. Is there a golden time after which there is no effect on the central nervous system?
6. Is there a correct does and treatment time for the hyperbaric oxygen?
7. Should there be repetitive treatments?
8. Are there cases of carbon monoxide poisoning that do not need to be treated with hyperbaric oxygen?

FUTURE STUDIES

We plan several protocols to delineate the effects of hyperbaric oxygen in modifying or preventing the encephalopathy associated wit CO poisoning. First we hope to determine if the <u>time interval</u> from the time of poisoning to the time of treatment is important, if there is <u>a dose</u> of CO tissue poisoning beyond which there is no reversal, and if there is the same relationship to <u>duration</u> of poisoning.

We plan to set protocols to determine the amount of oxygen necessary to treat the CO poisoning and the duration of the treatment which is necessary, if there is a reason to re-treat, and if so how long and how much.

SUMMARY

To date we have established an animal model with parameters to measure circulation, impaired circulation, shock, and tissue hypoxia.

Our animal model offers a methodology and measurement to evaluate the neuropathology associated with CO poisoning.

This animal model and methodology will hopefully delineate the roles of hyperbaric oxygen treatment of central nervous system poisoning by carbon monoxide.

REFERENCES

1. Takamatus I, Takeichi M, Yukitake A: Light and Electronicmicroscopic Observations on Brains of Experimentally Induced CO Poisoning in Cats. Adv. Neurol Sci (Japan) 13: 49-55, 1969.
2. Ginsberg MD, Myers RE: Experimental Carbon Monoxide Encephalopathy in the Primate. Arch Neurol 30: 202-216, March 1974.
3. Goldbaum LR, Ramirez G, Abalon KB: What is the Mechanism of Carbon Monoxide Toxicity? Aviat Space Environ Med 1289-1291, October 1975.
4. Ginsberg MD: Carbon Monoxide Intoxication Clinical Features Neuropathology and Mechanisms of Injury. Clinical Toxicology 23 (4-6): 281-288, 1985.
5. Fujii M: The Histopathology of the Central Nervous System Lesions Caused by Carbon Monoxide Poisoning. A Report of Ten Cases with an Acute and Protracted Clinical Course. Psychiatry Neurol (Japan) 62: 1-34, 1960.
6. Gorbon EB: CArbon Monoxide Encephalopathy. Br Med J i:1232, 1965.
7. Meyers RAM, Snyder SK, Emhoff TA: Subacute Sequelae of Carbon Monoxide Poisoning. Ann Emerg Med 14 (12): 1163-11267.
8. Kindwall EP: Hyperbaric Treatment of Carbon Monoxide Poisoning. Ann Emerg Med 14 (12) 1233-1234, December 1985.
9. NorKol DM: Treatment of Acute Carbon Monoxide Poisoning with Hyperbaric Oxygen. Ann Emerg Med 14 (12): 1168:1171, December 1985.
10. Mathieu D, Nolf M, Durocher A, Saulnier F, Frimat P, Furon D, Wattel F: Acute Carbon Monoxide Poisoning Risk of Late Sequelae and Treatment by Hyperbaric Oxygen. Clinical Toxicology 23 (4-6): 315-324, 1985.
11. Sawada, Yusuke, Ohashi N, Maemura K, Yoshioka T, Takahashi M, Fusamoto H, Kobayashi H, Suzimoto T: Computerized Tomography as an Indication of Long-Term Outcome After Acute Carbon Monoxide Poisoning. Lancet 783-784, April 12, 1980.
12. Ginsberg MD, Hedley-Whyte ET, Richardson EP: Hypoxic-Ischemic Leukoencepahlopathy in MAn. Arch Neurol 33:5-14, January 1986.

Hyperbaric oxygen therapy at 1.5 or 2.0 ATA as an adjunct to the rehabilitation of stabilized stroke patients

A controlled study

A. Marroni, Data P. G. * and Pilotti L.

Centro Iperbarico Policalente di Ricrca
S. Atto, Teramo, Italy
* Dept. of Physiology
University of Chieti
Chieti, Italy

INTRODUCTION

Hyperbaric Oxygen (HBO) has been used in the treatment of cerebral ischemia since 1961 (1-7) in the attempt to correct local hypoxia and to restore oxygen-dependent functions.

It is thought that in chronic stabilized stroke marginally functioning neurons may exist, receiving an amount of oxygen that can insure survival but not proper function. Restoring an appropriate oxygenation by HBO or revascularization procedures has been shown to improve functional and electrical cerebral activity (5,7,8,9); and HBO-induced improvement of cerebral function was used as a diagnostic tool for the suitability of revascularization surgical procedures even after intervals as long as 4 months or more after stroke (5,6,9).

The question of the most appropriate pressure of HBO for the treatment of neurological disorders is still debated by many Authors and most seem to favor pressures of 1.5 ATA. (10)

On the other hand it is known how well defined functional improvements may occur spontaneously or with appropriate physical therapy even after consistent intervals of time from stroke; it is therefore appropriate to think that the improvements observed with HBO treatments may be spontaneous and coincidental (11).

MATERIALS AND METHODS

80 stabilized stroke patients, all in possession of full clinical, angiographic and CAT-scan documentation proving the thrombotic nature of the

disease, and not any more undergoing any form of therapy or rehabilitation were selected for the study after obtaining informed consent. The patients, 55 males and 25 females, average age 59.7 yrs. (24-78), who had suffered from a stroke episode from 2 to 172 months before (average 29.2 months), were assigned to 8 study groups as follows:

A: Control group, not undergoing any form of treatment (8 males, 3 females, average age 60.8 yrs, average interval from stroke 31.6 mos. {3-107}).

B: Rehabilitation group, undergoing an in-water physical therapy protocol (12) during 30 sessions of 40 minutes duration in 30°Celsius water in our swimming pools. (5 males, 2 females, age 66.4 yrs. ave., interval from stroke 18 mos. ave. {2-46}).

C1: HBO group, undergoing 30 HBO sessions of 60 minutes at 2.0 ATA (8 males, 7 females, age 57 yrs ave., interval from stroke 42.9 mos. ave. {3-172}).

C2: HBO group, same as above but at 1.5 ATA pressure (6 males, 4 females, age 62.9 yrs. ave., interval from stroke 19.5 mos. ave. {6-72}).

D1: HBO and Rehabilitation group, undergoing HBO at 2.0 ATA in the afternoon and rehabilitation in the morning as above described (5 males, 4 females, age 60.4 yrs. ave., interval from stroke 47.2 mos. ave. {13-119}).

D2: HBO and Rehabilitation group as above - 1.5 ATA HBO (5 males, 2 females, age 63.7 yrs ave., interval from stroke 24.4 mos. ave. {3-107}).

E1: Hyperbaric Rehabilitation group, undergoing rehabilitation as above described during the course of the HBO sessions in our specially built "Hyperbaric Pool" at a water temperature of 30 Celsius, (11 males, 1 female, age 54.8 yrs. ave., interval from stroke 18.9 mos. ave. {5-42}).

E2: Hyperbaric Rehabilitation group as above - 1.5 ATA HBO (7 males, 2 females, age 51.5 yrs. ave., interval from stroke 31.2 mos. ave. {3-66}).

All HBO patients breathed oxygen via a BIBS mask-overboard dump system and were monitored for their arterial oxygen content at pressure to ensure the breathing of the desired oxygen tension.

The patients were evaluated by a neurologist, in a single blind fashion and according to a Neuromotor Disability Evaluation Scale, previously developed at our Center (13), which uses discrete, quantitized and repeatable ergometric indexes for ten groups of limb or system functions, summed up to a final score. Examples are finger and hand function, arm abduction, muscular strength, walking ability and speed, quality of gait.

The evaluations were performed on day 1, 10, 20, 30 of treatment and after 1 and 3 months after treatment. Every time the neuromotor disability score was computed and recorded without the knowledge of the precedently evaluated ones. At the end of the study the scores were confronted and the differential values compared to evaluation 1 were recorded for each patient and mediated for each group. The data were plotted and are reported in figures 1 and 2.

RESULTS

Control group A and Rehabilitation group B both showed an improvement of one degree in our scale by the end of the study, (a learning effect?). (fig.1).

All HBO groups showed more definite improvements in their neuromotor disability, but no significant difference could be noted amongst the four groups which scored from 3.1 to 3.8 degree improvements. (fig.1).

Both Hyperbaric Rehabilitation groups showed more distinct improvements, the 1.5 ATA group reaching 8.1 degree at 1 month after treatment and levelling off at 7.7 at 3 months, while the 2.0 ATA group showed a sharp 11.6 degree improvements which was still present 3 months after treatment. (fig.1).

The data were again elaborated and groups A-B and C1-C2-D1-D2 were averaged and plotted together (fig.2). It appears that although a well defined difference exists among the 4 groups in fig. 2 and all the HBO ones show distinct improvements, the only clearcut significant improvement was obtained by groups E1 and E2, the Hyperbaric Rehabilitation groups, and more markedly by group E1 (2.0 ATA HBO).

DISCUSSION

The physical activity involved in the HBO treatment given to the Hyperbaric Rehabilitation groups, together with an expectable counteraction of the warm water temperature towards the vasoconstrictive effect of HBO, may be in favor of an increased peripheral blood flow and an improved peripheral oxygenation.

According to Paulson (14), affected cerebral zones lose their circulatory autoregulation capacity, can resent general circulatory variations, and when confronted with a controlateral vasoconstriction, can show a paradoxic blood flow increase, the so called reverse steal phenomenon.

All this together may, theoretically and as it seems to appear from out data, be consistent with an improved circulation and cerebral blood flow in the affected brain areas, which might enhance local oxygenation in the presence of the highly favorable diffusion gradient provided by HBO. Considering the reverse steal phenomenon's possibility, the stronger vasoconstrictive effect of 2.0 ATA HBO might enhance local blood vasoconstrictive effect of 2.0 ATA HBO might enhance local blood flow in the affected brain area and give a higher diffusion gradient than 1.5. ATA HBO.

HBO alone, not associated with activity in warm water, might not similarly influence peripheral and local blood flow. Physical activity in warm water per se, on the other hand, while causing a similar peripheral and possibly cerebral blood flow effect, lacks the higher PAO2, the cerebral vasoconstriction and the possibility of a reverse steal phenomenon to provide extra oxygen to marginally functioning zones of the brain.

In conclusion, and looking only at the crude date, it appears that HBO treatment per se, as described in this study, associated or not with physical therapy performed in separate sessions, causes a certain improvement in the neuromotor performance of chronic stabilized stroke patients compared with similar patients in the Control and Rehabilitation groups. Standard deviations are anyway quite relevant and extremes overlap.

There appears to be no difference between treatment at 1.5 or 2.0 ATA Oxygen pressures, so 1.5 may be the choice in this cases.

HBO associated with simultaneous in water Rehabilitation - Hyperbaric Rehabilitation - as described in this study, appears to yield significant improvements in the neuromotor performance and general disability of stabilized stroke patients, especially as treatment pressures of 2.0 ATA.

ABSTRACT

HYPERBARIC OXYGEN THERAPY AT 1.5 OR 2.0 ATA AS AN ADJUNCT TO THE REHABILITATION OF STABILIZED STROKE PATIENTS. A CONTROLLED STUDY

Marroni A., Data P.G., Pilotti, L.

HBO Therapy has been studied by many Authors as an adjunctive treatment for stroke patients. Satisfactory results have been reported for the use of HBO as a predictive tool for EC-IC revascularization. The question of the appropriate treatment pressure has been debated in the literature.

We studied a group of 80 well stabilized cerebral thrombosis patients not any more undergoing any form of treatment or care. Average age was 59.7 yrs., average stroke age 29.2 months. The patients were divided into 8 groups: A: control group not undergoing any care; B: in water rehabilitation, 30 sessions, no HBO; C1: 30 HBO sessions at 2.0 ATA; C2: same at 1.5 ATA; D1: HBO at 2 ATA plus rehabilitation as above; D2: same at 1.5 ATA; E1: HBO and simultaneous Rehabilitation in our specially built Hyperbaric pool at 2 ATA; E2: same at 1.5. ATA

The Rehabilitation protocol was originally developed at our Center as well as a quantitized and repeatable Neuromotor Disability Evaluation Scale. Patients were controlled prior to beginning, every 10 days during treatment, then 1 and 3 months after.

Obtained data show defined and similar HBO effects on the improvement of patients' performance at 1.5 and 2.0 ATA, a clear and significant potentiation of this effect being evident for the Hyperbaric Rehabilitation groups and especially for the group treated at 2.0 ATA. The obtained results were still present at the third month after treatment.

Key words: HBO Therapy, Stroke, Rehabilitation, Neuromotor Disability Evaluation

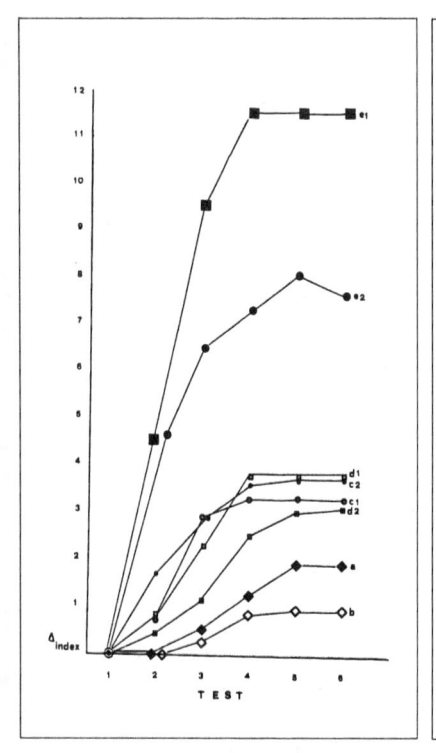

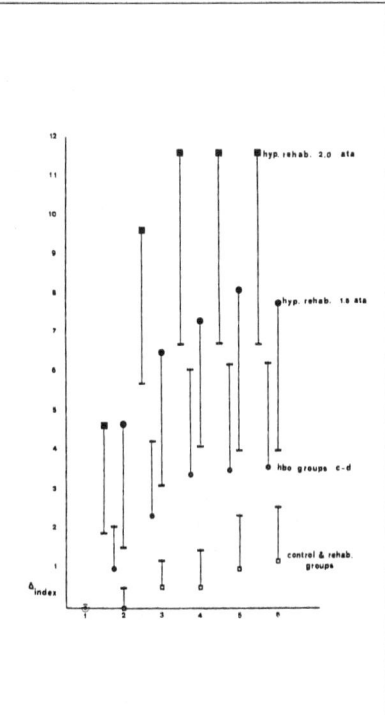

Figure 1. Mean improvement in neuromotor disability index in the different study groups - A: Control, B: In water rehabilitation, C1: HBO 2.0 ATA, C2: HBO 1.5 ATA, D1: HBO 2.0 ATA and in water rehabilitation, D2: HBO 1.5 ATA and in water rehabilitation, E1 AND E2: Hyperbaric in water rehabilitation breathing 2.0 and 1.5 ATA HBO. {See text}

Figure 2. Mean improvement in neuromotor disability index and S.D. values for hyperbaric rehabilitation at 1.5 and 2.0 ATA, HBO groups C and D {1.5 and 2.0 ATA}, control and rehabilitation groups. {See text}

REFERENCES

1. Smith G, Lawson D, Renfrew S, Preservation of Cerebral Cortical Activity by Breathing Oxygen at 2.0 ATA of Pressure during Cerebral Ischemia, Surg. Genecol. Obstet. 113: 13-16; 1961.
2. Sukoff MG, Hollin SA, Jacobsen JH, The Protective Effect of Hyperbaric Oxygenation in Experimentally Produced Cerebral Edema and Compression Surgery 62: 40-46; 1967.
3. Saltzman HA, Anderson B, Whalen RE, Hyperbaric Oxygen Therapy of Acute Cerebral Vascular Insufficiency, Proceedings of the 3rd International Conference on Hyperbaric Medicine. Nat. Acad. Nat. Res. Coucnil Publ. N 1401: 440-446; 1966.
4. Hart GB, Thompson RE, The treatment of Ischemia with Hyperbaric Oxygen, Strok 2: 296-300; 1971.
5. Holbach KH, Wassman H, Bonatelli AP, A Method to Identify and Treat Reversible Alterations of the Brain Tissue, In: Schmeidek P Ed., Microsurgery for Stroke. Springer Werlag , New York 1977
6. Kapp JP, Neurological Response To Hyperbaric Oxygen, a Criterion for Cerebral Revascularization, Surg. Neurol. 15: 43-46; 1981
7. Neubauer RA, Hyperbaric Oxygenation as an Adjunct Therapy in Strokes due to Thrombosis. A Review of 122 Patients, Stroke 11: 297-300; 1980
8. Symon L, The Concept of Threshold of Ischemia in Relation to Brain Structure and Function, J. Clin. Path. Suppl. 11: 149-154; 1976
9. Roski R, Spetzler RF, Owen H, Reversal of a Seven Year Old Visual Field Defect with EC-IC Arterianstomosis, Surg. Neurol. 10: 267-268; 1978
10. Holbach KH, Caroli A, Wassman H, Cerebral Energy Metabolism in Patients with Brain Lesions at Normo and Hyperbaric Oxygen Pressures, J. Neurol. 217: 17-30; 1977
11. Heimbach RD, Hyperbaric Oxygen Therapy and Stroke, JAMA 245: 1873-1874; 1981
12. Marroni A, Data PG, Pilotti L, Ossigeno Terapia Iperbarica e Fisioterapia in Vettore Umido nella Riabilitazione delle Lesioni Cerebro Vascolari Proceedings of the International Post-Graduate Course in Anesthesia and Intensive Care, Gismondi A, Caione R, Colonna S Eds. 479-516. Otranto, Italy, 15-22 June 1985. Editrice Salentina, Galatina, Italy
13. Marroni A, Data PG, Pilotti L, Hyperbaric Oxygen Therapy and In Water Rehabilitation for Chronic Stabilized Stroke Patients, Proceedings of the 1st Swiss Symposium on Hyperbaric Medicine 83-101, Basel 13-14 October 1986, J. Schmuntz Ed. Drager, Lubeck, Germany
14. Paulson in Neubauer RA, Hyperbaric Oxygen Therapy of Stroke. A Review, R.A. Neubauer, USA ISBN 0-9612512-0-4, Lib. Cong. Cat. Card N 83-90177; 1983

Acute hydrogen sulphide poisoning treated with hyperbaric oxygen

Peng Hsu, M.D.

Hyperbaric Oxygen Unit, Department of Surgery,
Rui Jin Hospital
Shanghai Second Medical University,
Shanghai, China

The author reports 10 cases of accidental exposure to H2S. Five of the victims died at the site of the exposure; the H2S concentration was still 600 mg/m3, four hours after the accident. Of the other five victims, four of them lost consciousness for two to 20 minutes with accompanying heart damage. One fell into deep coma and regained consciousness only after four treatments of HBO therapy within the ensuing 48 hours; heart, liver and renal damage were observed subsequently. All patients recovered uneventfully after HBO therapy or combination with the use of nitrites. Subsequent follow-up to date revealed no abnormality whatsoever.

CASE PRESENTATION

A male victim, aged 28, lost consciousness at the site of exposure at 9:30 a.m. on April 7, 1986. After a few minutes the victim was delivered to the emergency room of a local hospital. Artificial respiration was carried out on the way, his breath smelt of "rotten eggs." His pupils were 7mm and were unresponsive to light; blood pressure was 140/90mm Hg with a sinus tachycardia of 150 min. Chest examination was normal. Amyl nitrite by inhalation and supplemental oxygen were begun immediately upon arrival in the emergency room.

Treatment with fluid, together with energetic treatments and electrolytes, sodium bicarbonate, mannitol, cytochrome C, coenzyme A, citicoline, decadron and cefobid, was started simultaneously.

At 12 p.m. tracheotomy was done and a transient S-T segment depression in ECG was noted.

Then the comatose patient was transported to the HBO chamber of Rui Jin Hospital by ambulance. At 3:30 p.m. the victim was placed into the multiplace chamber with a physician and a trained nurse in attendance. The patient was treated with 100% oxygen at 2.5 ATA for 80 min. The ECG monitoring (Figs. 1,2) in the chamber revealed an increase in T wave amplitude which was still within normal range and the P wave became prominent with a notch on the ascending limb. After the first treatment of HBO, his eyeballs moved spontaneously. At 10:50 p.m. the second treatment of HBO was begun, and the patient started to response to stimuli. The third HBO treatment proceeded at 8:30 a.m., April 8, and the fourth was performed at 3:25 p.m. The patient became conscious gradually. On the morning of April 9, he recovered consciousness, answering questions coherently, and memory was recovered. A formal neurological examination disclosed no objective abnormality. On the third day after poisoning, BUN (Fig. 4) increased to 39.2 mg/dl and did not return to normal until the 13th day (8.2mg/dl). On the eighth day, SGPT (Fig. 5) was elevated to 108u (HBV tests were within normal range, the liver and the spleen were not enlarged). SGPT returned to normal (36u) on the 15th day. On the ninth day, EEG was almost normal. In the ECG studies, the P wave returned to normal on the 21st day and T wave on the 36th day (Figs. 1, 2).

DISCUSSION

H_2S is a highly toxic, inflammable, colorless gas, readily recognized in low concentration by its characteristic "rotten eggs" odor. The 10 victims reported in this paper exposed at the site of high concentration H_2S which was generated from the sewage. In general, when the concentration of H_2S approached $1000mg/m^3$, the victims may die suddenly. During the accident, the concentration of H_2S probably exceeded toxic levels (the concentration was still $600mg/m^3$ for four hours later). Hence, five victims died immediately after exposure. The signs and symptoms, especially those related to the CNS, are generally obvious after exposure to high concentrations of H_2S.

Burnett (1) reported 221 cases of H_2S poisoning and most of them experienced a period of unconsciousness, while 74% had a loss of consciousness at the accident site, and 16% in the emergency room.

In our five victims, four had a loss of consciousness for two to 20 minutes after exposure, while the other comatose patient became conscious after four treatments of HBO therapy were given in the ensuing 48 hours. In addition, the lungs are frequently affected, with 52% of the victims receiving some form of respiratory assistance, and 20% suffering from pulmonary edema (1). In our comatose patient, although tracheotomy was performed due to apnea in the emergency room, no pulmonary edema occurred from the beginning to the end.

ECG monitoring showed T wave change in all five victims. In one of the five, ECG showed an increased amplitude of the T wave in II, III, AVF, V3, V5, not correlated to the blood serum K concentration (Fig. 3). In II, III and V5, the P wave became prominent with a notch on the ascending limb. The former might be due to myocardial hypoxia, while the latter is due to H_2S intoxication which caused spasm as well as an increase in blood pressure in the pulmonary arteriole.

The liver and kidney damage in the most severe patient, as revealed by a short period of elevation in SGPT and BUN, could not be explained by other causes such as antibiotics, hepatitis or other drugs.

Burnett reported a BUN concentration from 11-170 mg/dl in 23 cases. Liver function tests were done in only 30% of the patients and abnormalities of enzyme concentrations were seen in several of the patients.

Sulphide ions act as direct cytotoxins, binding selectively to cytochrome oxidase within the mitochondria and thereby disrupting the electron transport chain, causing cell anoxia, especially in the CNS.

In theory, nitrites aid the conversion of hemoglobin to methemoglobin, the latter, by binding free sulphide ions, spares intracellular cytochrome oxidase. Amyl nitrite pearls for inhalation induce methemoglobin which competes with the cytochrome system for the sulphide ions by forming sulphide methemoglobin (Fig. 7). Although this mode of therapy has been suggested in literature, controversies still exist as to its beneficial use.

THE ROLE OF HBO IN TREATMENT OF H2S POISONING

HBO therapy for H2S poisoning is still in the stage of experimental investigation.

We speculate that mechanisms of HBO (Fig. 6) used in H2S poisoning benefits hyperoxygenation, vasoconstriction, edema reduction and oxygen diffusion in the brain tissue, as well as the protection of other vital organs such as heart, liver and kidney from the hypoxia initiated by H2S intoxication.

In the experimentation of Talmi (1) et al., intoxication was produced in 100 rats, by the injection of Sodium Sulphide intraperitoneally (55 mg/kg). The animals were divided into five groups: 1) controls - without treatment; 2) sodium nitrite treatment (60 mg/kg I.P.); 3) treated by 100% oxygen; 4) treated by 3 ATA oxygen for 60 min.; and 5) sodium nitrite treatment together with 3ATA oxygen. Significant improvement in treatment with 3 ATA oxygen and the combined treatment of oxygen + nitrites, as indicated by the survival rates, was proved using the Fisher exact-test ($P<0.005$). Dramatic improvement was seen in the EEG of poisoned rats during exposure to hyperbaric oxygen.

For the four moderate and one severe cases, 11 and 15 treatments of HBO therapy had been given respectively. All five patients recovered uneventfully after HBO therapy or combination with the use of nitrites. Subsequent follow-up to date revealed no abnormality whatsoever. Our results suggest that HBO is an effective treatment for acute H2S intoxication and should be instituted as soon as possible.

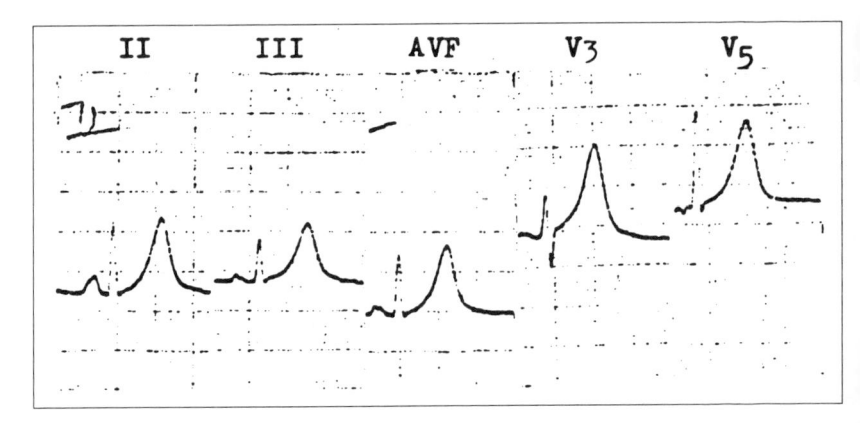

Figure 1. A comatose victim, male, aged 28, accident on April 7, 1986. EGC showed an increased amplitude in the T wave. (Returned to normal on 36th day.)

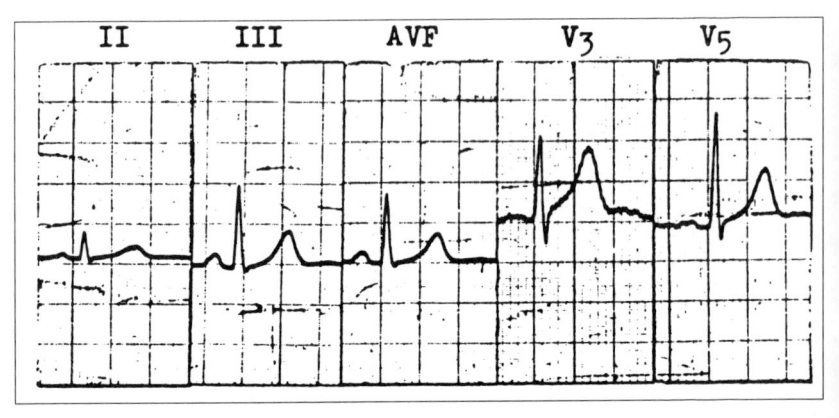

Subsequent follow-up to date no abnormality.

133

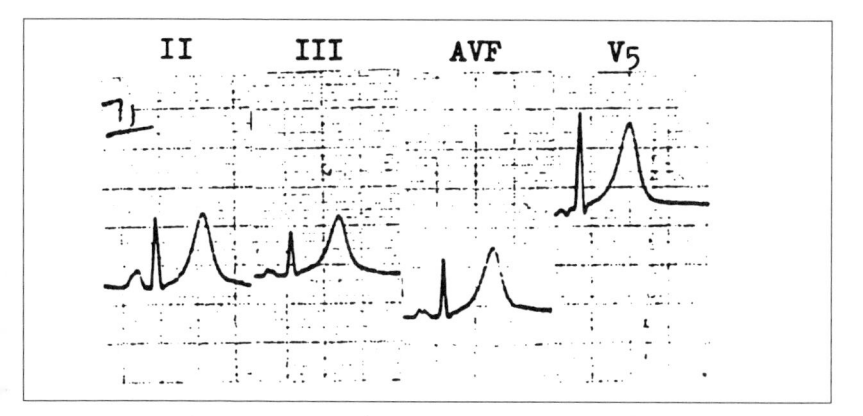

Figure 2. Same victim, P wave became prominent with a notch on ascending limb.

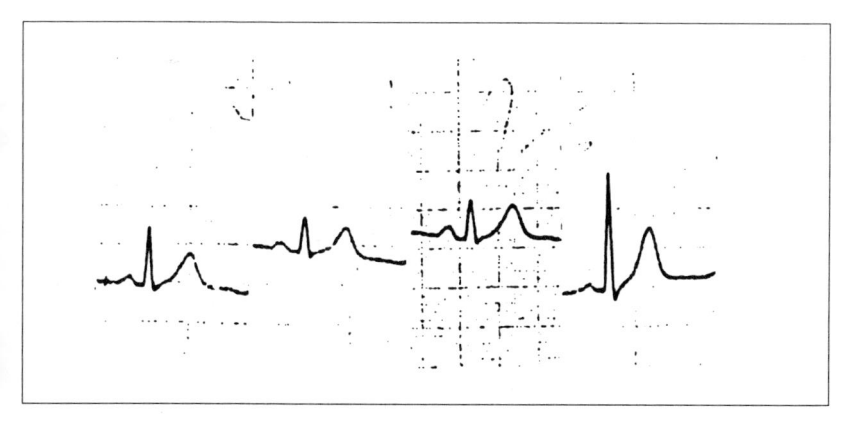

Returned to normal on 21st day.

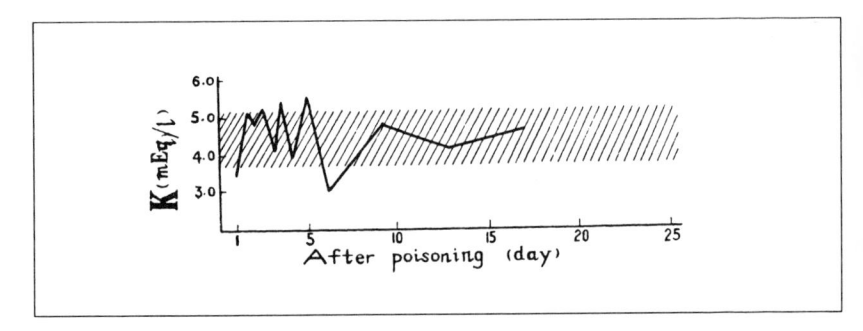

Figure 3. A male victim, age 28, comatose, blood serum K concentration observed within normal range, were not correlated with ECG monitoring revealed an increase in T wave amplitude.

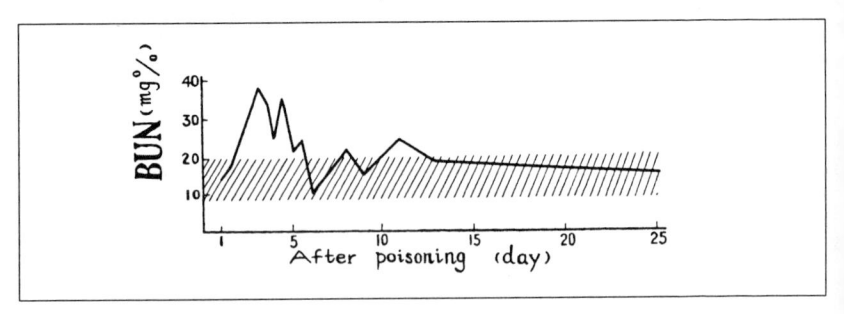

Figure 4. Same victim, on 3rd day after poisoning. BUN increased to 39.2mg/dl and returned to normal 18.2mg/dl on the 13th day.

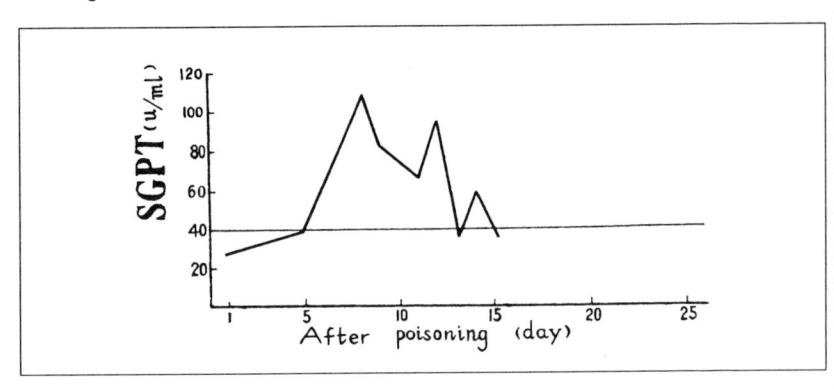

Figure 5. Same victim, SGPT elevated to 108u on the 8th day and returned to normal 36u on the 15th day.

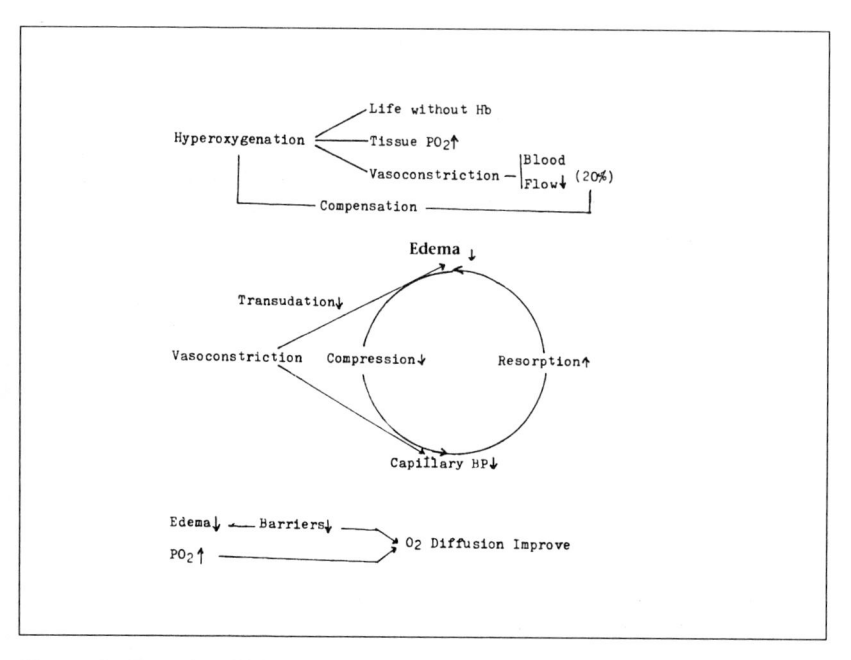

Figure 6. Postulated Mechaniam of HBO.

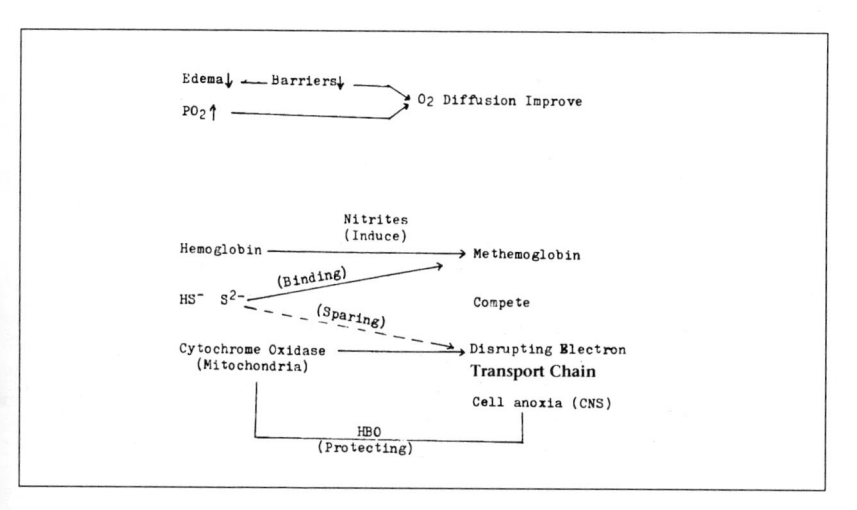

Figure 7. Scheme of Role of HBO and Nitrites in Acute H_2S Poisoning.

REFERENCES

1. Burnett WW et al.: Hydrogen sulfide poisoning: Review of 5 years' experience. Can Med Asso J 117: 1277, 1977.
2. Talmi Y et al.: Hyperbaric oxygen therapy in experimental acute sulfide poisoning in rats. In: Program and Abstracts, XI Annual Meeting of EUBS on Diving and Hyperbaric Medicine, Goteborg, Sweden, 21-23 Aug. 1985, p.15.

The ARMS experience of hyperbaric oxygen therapy for multiple sclerosis

D. J. D. Perrins and P.B. James

Honorary Advisers in Hyperbaric Medicine to ARMS.
4a Chapel Hill, Stansted, Essex CM24 8AG,
United Kingdom

Action for Research into Multiple Sclerosis (ARMS) is a British charity and was founded in 1975 by people with MS who wished to participate in research projects concerned with the cause, diagnosis, prevention and treatment of the condition.

The early reports of a beneficial effect of HBO, and Fisher's controlled trial at New York University (1), induced ARMS to conduct a small confirmatory study in Dundee (2). The improvements experienced by their members there persuaded them, in 1983, to make the treatment available throughout the United Kingdom.

Fifty-two Centres are now operational (Fig. 1) and most are equipped with purpose-built, single lock, chambers that accommodate six or more people. They are staffed by salaried managers and volunteer assistants (usually patient's relatives) who have been trained and supervised by ARMS Staff. The patients are invited to make a donation towards the cost of each treatment - about £5 ($7[m] US).

Most patients refer themselves or are brought by their relatives. It is clearly explained that they may receive no benefit, and even if they do, not all symptoms will respond. Family doctors are asked to assent to their patient receiving hyperbaric oxygen therapy.

In the early days a pressure of 2.0 ATA was routinely employed but some patients complained that their symptoms were exacerbated. It was then found that lower pressures were effective so that it is now the practice to start a course of daily treatments at 1.25 ATA for one hour when, after 20 daily sessions, about 30% show signs of improvement on, or about, the fourth day. Those who do not respond after five sessions are then taken to 1.5 ATA, when a further 50% respond.

The rest nearly all improve at 1.75 ATA, though very occasionally 2.0 ATA does have to be employed.

Each Centre obtains essentially the same results which compare with those from the earlier reports; fatigue, bladder, balance and speech symptoms responding particularly well. Such improvements are often lost within a week or two but are immediately restored by only one exposure to the pressure at which they had previously responded. The need for regular maintenance doses is obvious, so patients are advised to attend for regular "top-ups" of an hour at least once a month, though some find that they have to return sooner. A few manage without for much longer.

The problems associated with the evaluation of any treatment for MS are well recognized and chiefly concern the spontaneous improvements that may occur and the inconsistency of methods for clinical assessment. The topic has been reviewed by Shumacher (3) who considers that satisfactory methods for conducting controlled trails to assess the effectiveness of any treatment have yet to be devised. He suggests that the sole criterion of efficacy should be the prevention of further downhill progression over a two year period, while any improvements are simply recorded as a failure to get worse. To this end, ARMS have trained suitable volunteers to assess each patient before, during and immediately after the initial course of treatment and to follow subsequent progress.

The ARMS Centre in Glasgow was the first to report their results. Seventy percent of 128 patients had responded to the initial course of 20 sessions and were reassessed a year later when two-thirds of those who had continued treatment had not deteriorated (Table 1).

This result may indicate the value of long-term treatment, but a controlled trial is necessary to exclude the possibility that patients only chose to continue with maintenance treatment if their condition was static or improving.

It is unreasonable to ask patients to volunteer to act as "double blind controls" and attend for possibly "dummy" treatment once a week for two years. However a valid study can be conducted retrospectively when patients are allocated at random either to either a "treated" or "control" group. A "treated" group can be patients who have completed regular follow-on sessions, while the patients who have completed regular follow-on sessions, while the "control" group can be those who have only received the initial series of 20 sessions. On breaking the code, those patients found not to have followed the group protocol to which they have been assigned are discarded from the study.

A study of this type was conducted in Oxford and revealed a considerable difference in the stability of "treated" and "control" groups when assessed at a year (Table 2).

Several other Centres have now been treating patients for two or more years and are beginning to submit their returns for computer analysis. A superficial scan of the initial printout suggests that the pattern continues to be followed; 78 patients from 10 Centres received weekly maintenance treatment for two years and 82% have not deteriorated, while 45% of 33 patients who did not attend after the initial course are significantly worse.

It should be appreciated that this report represents early work but indicates that it should continue.

Table 1. Condition of 128 patients in Glasgow a year after an initial course of HBO.

	Stable	Deteriorated
Regular "booster" sessions (1 or more every 5 weeks)	4	22
No maintenance	13	32
		= <0.001

Table 2. The Oxford results from 62 patients randomly allocated to receive regular maintenance treatment or to act as controls.

	62 patients Random allocation	
	Regular maintenance	No maintenance
	31	31
Complied with their allocation	18	12
Stable at one year	15 (83%)	1 (8%)

Table 3. Long term results in Guernsey centre.

	2 Years 47 patients	3 Years 26 patients
Improved	65%	46%
Stable	26%	44%
Deteriorated	10%	10%

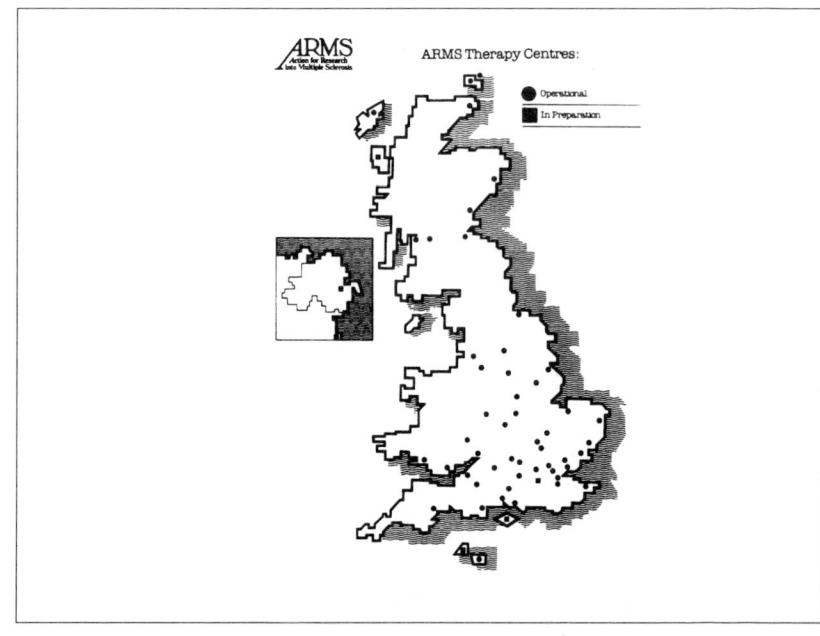

Figure 1. The location of the Centres.

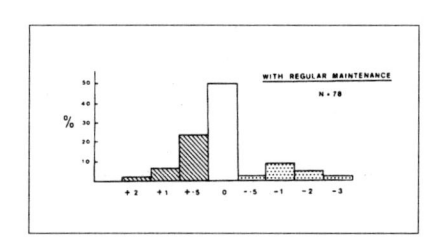

REFERENCES
1. Fischer BH, Marks M, Reich T. Hyperbaric-oxygen treatment of multiple sclerosis: a randomized, placebo-controlled, double blind study. N Eng J Med 1983; 308: 181-186.
2. Davidson DLW. Hyperbaric oxygen treatment for multiple sclerosis. Practitioner 1984; 228: 903-905.
3. Schumacher GA. Critique of experimental trials of therapy in multiple sclerosis. Neurology 1974; 24: 1010-1014.

The severe fat embolism treated by the combination therapy using hyperbaric oxygen and conventional methods

Hiroshi Yagi
Fukuoka Yagi Kosei-kai Hospital

Mitsuko Ohshima
Fukuoka Yage Kosei-kai Hospital and
Second Dept. of Internal Medicine
Faculty of Medicine, Kyushu Univ.

Toshihiro Toyonaga
Dept. of Orthopedic Surgery
Faculty of Medicine, Kyushu Univ.

Toshiro Yanai
Second Dept. of Internal Medicine
Faculty of Medicine, Kyushu Univ.

Shozo Sadoshima
Second Dept. of Internal Medicine
Faculty of Medicine, Kyushu Univ.

Hitoshi Fukui
Dept. of Neuro-Surgery
Faculty of Medicine, Kyushu Univ.
Fukuoka, Japan

INTRODUCTION

Most of subclinical systemic fat embolism occur after long bone fractures, and in Japan only one or two percent of the incidence of the clinically apparent fat embolism syndrome of the fracture cases has been reported [1]. The mechanism producing fat embolism syndrome (FES) which are hypoxia, confusion and petechiae, is still not clearly explained. It is considered, however, that the hypoxia due to the fat particles released in the lesion is one of the most important factors of producing FES.

From this understanding, we have employed the hyperbaric oxygen (HBO) for these cases together with the conventional medical therapies, and we have treated 5 of the clinically apparent cases occurring within 24 hours after long bone fractures.

METHODS AND SUBJECT

For the treatment of the FES cases, the HBO therapy using multiplace chamber (Kawasaki Engineering Co. KHO301) was performed under the condition of 2ATA for 90 minutes once a day, and in accordance with patients's conditions 3 to 30 times exposures of HBO were given. Physical and neurological examinations were given every day, and the consciousness was graded according to the following classifications. That is, the grade 0 is normal, the grade I is the condition in which a case awakes without stimulus, the grade II is that a case is awaked by stimulus and the III is that a case is not awaked by stimulus. The examinations of CT, EEG, blood gas analysis and chest X-ray were performed a few times depending on patients' conditions, and Hb, thrombocyte, serum albumin and cardiothoracic ratio (CTR) were also measured.

For the cases with the delayed impaired consciousness and speech disturbance after recovering from coma, 2 mg/day of thyrotropin releasing hormone tartrate (TRH-T) was given intravenously with HBO therapy. Latency time from the injury to the onset was estimated based on the notes from the physicians and/or nurses.

During about 9 years from Jan. 1 1978 to Nov. 30, 1986, 193 and 400 cases of upper and lower extremities respectively with long bone fractures were treated in Yagi Kosei-kai Hospital. 53 cases of the multiple fractures were found in them.

All of our 5 cases with the clinically apparent FES has long bone fractures of lower extremity, and 2 cases of them also had the fractures of upper extremity. Three out of our FES 5 cases were transferred to our hospital (transferred case) after post traumatic neurological deterioration had appeared and neurosurgeons had diagnosed these cases fat embolism. Another 2 cases were primarily examined in our hospital immediately after the injury (nontransferred case).

All cases of FES had the femoral bone fractures. 4 of them received the wire extension and the other 1 case received intramedullary fixation for the single fracture of the femur after the injury. The incidence of fat embolism was 0.84% in 593 fracture cases, however, it showed 7.55% in 53 multiple fracture cases.

Age distribution was from 16 to 37 years, 23.4 years on an average in young men.

RESULTS

In 3 transferred cases, 2 were in the condition of coma, and the other 1 case was in semicoma when they had been carried to our hospital. Estimated latency time of the transferred cases from the injury to the onset of FES was 13, 24 and 12 hours respectively. On the other hand, 2 nontransferred cases had respiratory insufficiency followed by coma or stupor within 1 hour, and the estimated latency time was 13 and 10 hours respectively.

For 2 nontransferred cases HBO therapy was performed immediately after the onset, and for 3 transferred cases the same therapy was performed as soon as they had been carried to our hospital after 24, 48 and 60 hours from the onset.

Before HBO, PaO_2 of 2 nontransferred cases was 41.0 and 38.5mmHg and $PaCO_2$ was 28.3 and 26.7mmHg respectively in room air. On the other hand, PaO_2 of 3 transferred cases was 67.0, 69.0 and 79.6mmHg and $PaCO_2$ was 29.0, 31.8 and 33.9mmHg respectively before HBO therapy. Hypoxia before HBO therapy of the nontransferred cases was more severe than that in the transferred cases.

During the HBO therapy, their PaO_2 increased over 700mmHg, but PaCO2 was constant.

The condition in each stuporous or semicomatose case was recovered after one or two exposures of HBO. On the contrary, the coma condition of 3 cases was not satisfactorily recovered even after 10 exposures, but verbal response was noticed (Tab. 1).

Clinical courses of the 3 cases fallen into coma were almost the same. That is, decorticate position was observed through the whole period of coma, and anisocoria and conjugated deviation were also found during 2 or 3 days after the onset. After 20 exposures of HBO, the delayed impaired consciousness and speech disturbance still remained, and then 2mg/day of TRH-T was given intravenously with HBO therapy for 10 days. As a result, they got rid of the consciousness and speech disturbance.

It was understood that the disturbance of consciousness tended to be more rapidly recovered when the patients received HBO therapy in earlier stage after the onset (Fig.1).

Any focal intracranial lesion except slight edema were not found by CT examination, though severely abnormal EEG mixed !!!!!!! and !!!!! waves was shown on the record in the whole area of the brain of 3 cases in coma. Pneumonia like shadow was observed in either side of the lung of all cases in the chest X-ray film. In 2 out of 3 transferred cases, the shadow was slight.

Our cases were diagnosed as FES according to Tsuruta's criteria. As for 3 major signs of FES, hypoxia, confusion and petechiae, in our cases the former 2 signs were observed, but petechiae were not observed.

As the medium signs of FES, PaO_2 below 70mmHg and Hb. below 10g/dL were demonstrated in 4 and 3 cases respectively, and moreover, as the minor signs, tachycardia over 120/min., fever over 38°C, thrymbocytopenia and hypo-albuminemia were observed in 4, 4, 2 and 2 cases respectively.

In order to prevent the release of the fat particle in the lesions, surgical repositions of fractured bones should be performed as soon as possible. Therefore, primary operation was done under the condition of coma. All of our cases were cured and have survived by the combination therapies of HBO and conventional treatment including cortico-steroid, and all patients have not had neurological deficits so far.

In retrospective studies, cardio-thoracic ratio (CTR) rather rapidly increased during 1 week after the onset, and after that it decreased gradually. On the other hand, the remarkable increase of CTR was not found in the cases of subclinical fat embolism.

DISCUSSION AND CONCLUSION

The number of the reports on fat embolism syndrome (FES) has recently been increased, the syndrome, however, is still rare occurrence in Japan [1].

The lucid interval between the injury and the onset is usually about 48 hours, however, the estimated latency time in our 5 cases were from 10 to 24 hours after the injury, 14.4 hours on an average. Our 5 cases were considered to be severe fat embolism because of the early onset of FES, and all cases had respiratory insufficiency followed by mental confusion. Therefore, hypoxia was considered to be one of the preferential factors which produce FES. However, the coma-condition of 1 nontransferred and 2 transferred cases was not recovered even though HBO therapy was given during about 10 days.

From the viewpoint of the results, we believe that the causes of post traumatic encephalophathy without head trauma might be resulted from both factors of hypoxia and multiple micro embolii in the brain, and CT examination couldn't detect them.

The mortality of post traumatic encephalopathy due to fat embolism has been reported [2] as high as 29% in the cases treated by conventional therapies alone, but all of our 5 cases treated by the combination therapy of HBO and conventional methods were cured and have survived over 2 years without any permanent deficits.

Through our results, it is suggested that the earlier the HBO therapy is performed, the more rapid recovery from the disturbance of consciousness may be expected.

Table 1.

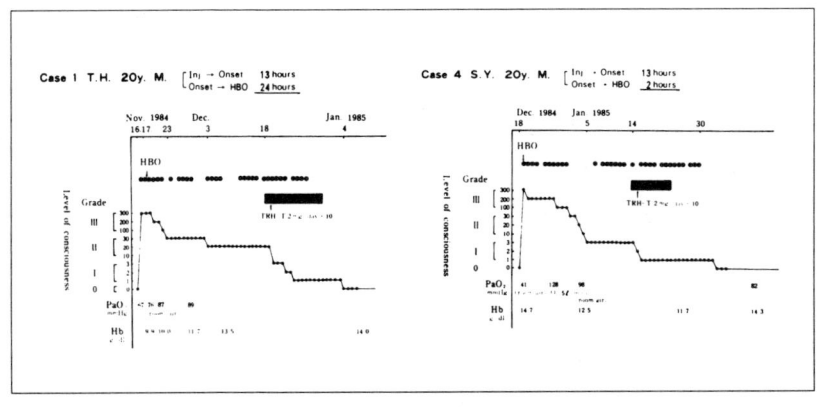

Figure 1.

REFERENCES

1. Tsuruta, T., Shiokawa, Y.; Fat Embolism, Seikei-geka Mook Vol. 5, P. 172-184, Kanehara Publisher, Tokyo, 1978.
2. Jacobson, D.M., Terrence, C.F. and Reinmuth, O.M.; The Neurological Manifestations of Fat Embolism. Neurology, 36: 847-851, 1986.

Hyberbaric lung lavage in pulmonary alveolar proteinosis

J.A.K. Peper, D.J. Bakker, C.M. Roos,, J.J. Schreuder, W.W.A. Zuurmond and H.M. Jansen

Academic Medical Center
University of Amsterdam
Meibergdreef 9
1105 AZ Amsterdam
The Netherlands

INTRODUCTION

Pulmonary Alveolar Proteinosis is a rare disease. The diagnosis is based upon histological finding: proteinaceous substances and carbohydrates are found in groups of alveoli, in adjacent distal airspaces and in small airways.

The symptoms may vary from fatigue and coughing to shortness of breath at rest and cyanosis.

Most pulmonary function tests will show decreased values. The chest X-ray shows a radiating feathery soft density resembling the pattern seen in pulmonary edema.

There is no specific treatment: antibiotics, steroids and expectorants have been used but no treatment proved to be superior. If there is no response to treatment and spontaneous remission does not occur, the patient may die from hypoxaemia.

Broncho alveolar lavage has proved to be an effective symptomatic treatment for Pulmonary Alveolar Proteinosis.

However, it may be impossible to perform whole lung lavages in patients with severe respiratory failure because of oxygenation through one lung might not be sufficient. Hyperbaric ventilation is a rational way to improve oxygenation by enhancing oxygen transport through the alveolar membrane. The lavaging procedure requires extensive monitoring because of the risk of aggravating hypoxaemia during one lung ventilation.

METHODS

Up till now 6 sessions of massive unilateral broncho-alveolar lavages under hyperbaric conditions have been performed n 3 patients. The patients were anesthetized with Etomidate, Fentanyl and Pancuronium. The were intubated with a left double lumen tube and ventilated with 100% oxygen. Anesthesia was maintained by continuous infusion of Etomidate and Fentanyl.

Monitoring consisted of EKG and heart rate, systemic arterial blood pressure, temperature, urine production, right arterial pressure (RAP), pulmonary artery pressure (PAP), pulmonary capillary wedge pressure, respiratory pressure (Presp), inspired oxygen concentration (FIO_2), expired carbondioxide concentration ($ETCO_2$), lung fluid filling pressure (Pfill) and in-chamber mixed venous oxygen saturation ($SatvO_2$) by fibre-optic technique.

The patients were placed in lateral position so that the lung to be lavaged was below. The chamber was pressurized up to 2 bar and the lung to be lavaged was blocked. The lung was filled via a tube with unbuffered NaCl 0.9% at 37°C starting with a volume of about its functional residual capacity. Ventilation was maintained by 100% oxygen through the other lung with tidal volume and ventilatory rate adjusted to maintain arterial carbon dioxide tensions ($PaCO_2$) between 35-55 mm Hg.

Lavage was performed by filling the lung with a hydostatic pressure up to 30 cm H_2O and emptying with moderate suction.

The volumes of lavage fluid used were not fixed but variable. The determining factors of the volumes were the (continuously monitored) Pfill, Presp and $SatvO_2$. A steep increase in Pfill or Presp, or a decrease in $SatvO_2$ was used as indication to stop filling. In this way we tried to prevent leakage into the ventilated lung.

The protein concentration in the effluent fluid samples was analyzed immediately. Lavaging was repeated until low protein levels were reached. When the lung lavage was completed the ventilated lung was blocked and the wet lung ventilated with 100% oxygen. An end-expiratory pressure of 10 cm H_2O was applied to establish lung expansion without distending the dry lung.

After 10 minutes both lungs were ventilated and the chamber was depressurized. Once the systemic arterial oxygen tensions (PaO_2) and $PaCO_2$ were adequate the patient was allowed to breathe spontaneously. Anesthesia was discontinued and after extubation the patient was allowed to breathe oxygen enriched air by mask.

RESULTS

To investigate the influence of the hyperbaric pressure on lungs with severe respiratory disturbances we compared (fig. 1) the PaO_2 at 1 and 2 bar in the three patients before their left and right lung lavage sessions. At a chamber pressure of 2 bar the PaO_2 was increased compared to that at 1 bar.

Throughout each lavage session we also observed a slow but continuous increase in PaO_2 and in mixed venous oxygen tension (PvO_2). Therefore we could reduce the FIO_2 gradually from 1.0 to 0.5 without jeopardizing the patient. This way the PaO$_2$ mostly remained below 500 mm Hg, a level of which we suppose will avoid oxygen toxicity during the 4 to 5 hours of exposure to oxygen.

Superimposed on the gradual increase of PaO$_2$ during the lavage procedure a fluctuation concomitant with emptying and filling of the lung was obvious. In fig. 2 the PaO$_2$ is plotted at these specific moments in each of the 6 lavages. This demonstrates an increase in PaO$_2$ during the fluid filling phase. The SatvO$_2$ paralleled these increasing oxygen tensions. Possible the hydrostatic filling pressure in the non-ventilated lung obstructs gradually the pulmonary capillary flow. This decrease in lung shunting may result in a better oxygenation.

During one of the filling phases patient C showed suddenly deteriorating changes. A higher Presp, lower ETCO$_2$, higher PAP and RAP and a decrease in systemic arterial blood pressure was recorded. The SatvO$_2$ did not increase during the filling phase as was expected. Therefore we decided to interrupt the filling of the lung. Since 500 ml out of 750 ml lavage fluid had disappeared we assumed leakage into the ventilated lung, causing impaired ventilation. By increasing the FIO$_2$ to 1.0 and suction of the ventilated lung life-threatening hypoxaemia was prevented. Subsequently all variable returned to baseline values.

We did not observe any consistent increase in RAP or PAP nor did urine production suggest fluid absorption from the lavaged lung into the circulation.

To investigate the reliability of continuous in-chamber SatvO$_2$ measurements, we compared values obtained in the chamber to those measure outside. There was a good correlation (R = 0.847).

To establish the overall effects of the broncho-alveolar lavages we measured pulmonary functions and blood gas tensions before the first lavage, 1 week after the left lung lavage, 1 week after the right lavage, then after half a year. Total lung capacity improved in 2 patients from 3.4 to 4.7 to 5.4 and 6.1 L respectively, whereas vital capacity rose from 2.7 and 3.3 to 3.9 and 4.1 L.

The carbon monoxide transfer factor corrected for hemoglobin content as a measurement for diffusion capacity improved from 23, 39 and 31 to 58, 98 and 35% respectively of the predicted normal value.

The PaO$_2$ rose in the 3 patients breathing room air from resp. 44, 57 and 59 to 76, 85 and 70 mm Hg.

The right-to-left shunting decreased from 26, 22 and 19% of the cardiac output to 13, 4.3 and 10% respectively. Chest X-ray showed clearing of the densities.

Examining the one year results, patient B seems to follow the expected clinical course since his pulmonary function is slowly declining. However, patients A and C are steadily improving without treatment. This remarkable delay in deterioration of patients A and C after the lavage assumes a phenomenon yet to be clarified.

CONCLUSION

Massive broncho-alveolar lavage improves the course of Pulmonary Alveolar Proteinosis. In case of severe respiratory failure hyperbaric ventilation will facilitate unilateral lavage. Intensive monitoring may provide that extra safety which will permit a more effective and safe lavage.

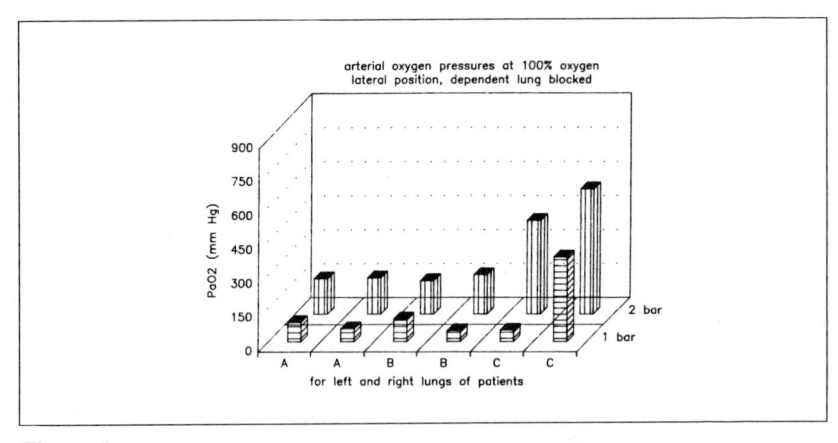

Figure 1.

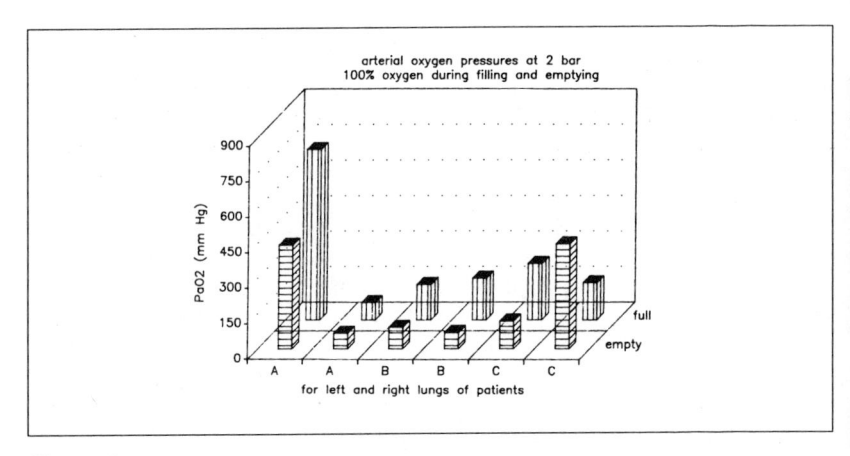

Figure 2.

HBO treatment of gastric and duodenal ulcers

Efuni S. N., Pogromov A. P., Egorov A. P. and Charayan L. V.

National Research Centre of Surgery, 1st Moscow Medical
Institute named by Sechenov, Moscow, USSR

In physiological conditions the resistance of the mucous membrane of the stomach and duodenum is regulated by 3 major interrelated mechanisms, they are mucus secretion, epithelium regeneration and adequate blood circulation. The failure of one of them destroys the whole defense mechanism that may result in ulcer formation.

There is an evidence that hypoxia and mucus hypoergosis might provoke gastric and duodenal ulcer formation. Thus, the therapy measures should be aimed at the restoration of metabolic processes activity in mucus membrane and duodenum. According to the modern views one of these treatments might be HBO which leads not only to oxygen metabolism restoration but also the normalization of cellular energy balance. HBO may activate biosynthetic and reparative processes in tissue.

This effect was illustrated by our research of acetate ulcers healing in rats (Okaba model) under the influence of HBO (regime of 2 ata for 45 min.). The results of the research were the following. (Fig. 1).

After 10 sessions of HBO (14th day following the initiation of the treatment, 24th day following the injury) the morphologic study of mucosal membrane of rats showed marked decrease in the size of fibrinoid necrosis zone as compared to the Control Group. Nectrotic masses layer was much thinner than in control animals. The extension of regenerating mucus was increased. We have studied the number of DNA of synthesized cells with thymidine, labeled with tririum. It was revealed that the label index increased threefold as compared to the Control Group. In some cases after the sessions of HBO ulcer healing was observed (there was not such a phenomena in the Control Group).

After 15 sessions of HBO (21 days following the initiation of the treatment, 31 days following the injury) ulcer healing was observed in some 60% of cases, in the Control Group of animals there was spontaneous scarforming process in some 20%. In those cases when after 15 sessions ulcers still remain their size is approximately 3 times smaller than in Control Group, they also do not have necrotic masses. Acetate stomach ulcers treated with 15 sessions of HBO have very specific features - in the new mucus membrane except for the mucus glands fundal glands containing parietal cells appear.

The data obtained proved the positive effect of HBO on chronic gastric ulcers healing in rats. This is manifested in more rapid disappearance of necrotic masses and enhancement of both stages of regeneration - proliferation and differentiation of epithelic cells of the gastric mucus membrane. The effect of HBO on the enhancement of regenerating processes was another important reason to include the said method into the modern anti-ulcer therapy.

217 patients (155 male and 62 female) with ulcer aged from 17 to 68 years were treated with HBO. Of these were 74 gastric ulcers and 143 duodenal ulcers. The majority of patients were treated in large therapeutic chamber of the National Centre of HBO with the regime of 1.72 ata, time of exposure - 45 min., compression and decompression time - 10 min. each. The drug therapy included as a rule only antacids - aluminum salts. But by the end of the 1st week of HBO treatment the patients needed no medicines any more. In most patients with gastric ulcer healing was 24.6 ± 1.8 days and of duodenal ulcer healing - 19.3 ± 0.37 days. Successful scar-forming process was observed along with quick regression of clinical symptoms if the disease. Hence in patients with duodenal ulcers nocturnal pains subsided after 2-3 sessions. Practically by the 7th - 9th HBO session complete pain relief was obtained and some time later dyspepsia signs disappeared. In the overwhelming majority of patients clinically ulcerous crisis was no longer observed by the 9th - 12th HBO sessions. The treatment efficacy was assessed by the endoscopic examination.

We consider the results of the treatment for the patients with persistent ulcers (more than 60 days) to be most important. In these patients the drug therapy in the preceding period included most up-to-date anti-ulcerous medicines: H2 - blockers of histamine receptors, drugs stabilizing mucus production (sucralfat, pollymoline, colloid vismute salts), regenerators (carbenoxiolole, solcoseryle), etc. (Fig. 2).

Nevertheless, it was not possible to obtain ulcer healing for a long period of time that is why the HBO treatment was initiated for these patients. The number of patients with persistent ulcers in the examination group comprised 39.2%, in some patients ulcer did not heal for a year or even longer. The routine HBO treatment gave promising results. Mean time of gastric and duodenal ulcers healing did not increase the time of treatment in the whole group of patients (gastric ulcer healing - 23.2 + 0.8 days, duodenal ulcer healing - 21.4 - 0.7 days). Such results allow us to recommend HBO as an additional conservative method of treatment. It is particularly indicated for the patients refusing surgery.

We have studied the results of ulcer treatment with HBO and modern anti-ulcerous drugs of various groups. The main group comprised 217 patients with ulcers treated with HBO, Control Group consisted of 350 patients treated with various drugs.

The reported results show that HBO method for the patients with ulcers may be a successful alternative or additional method used in modern anti-ulcerous therapy.

Intragastric pH-metry performed during the session revealed the decrease in basal level of acidity production mainly during decompression. The restoration of the initial level of intragastric pH by the end of the session was observed only in several patients. The decrease in the secretion level was accompanied by the drop in histamine concentration in peripheral blood and improvement of gastric acido-neutrolising function.

According to this criteria the changes in gastric secretion affected by HBO should be viewed separately in several groups of patients with ulcer and chronic gastritis: 1 - Gastric ulcer with initially normal or initially decreased secretion, 2 - Ulcer duodenum with normal or initially increased secretion, 3 - Chronic focal atrophic gastritis with hypochlorhydria, 4 - Chronic diffusive astrophic gastritis with histamine-resistant achlorhydria. (Fig. 3).

The conducted studies showed that in Group 1 after HBO therapy course hour volume of gastric secretion and discharge/hour of free HCL discharge both at the basal and stimulated stages of secretion is increased. In the majority of patients the level of free HCL discharge at the stimulated stage is restored to the normal level. In patients with ulcer located in pyloroduodenal zone the changes in the studied parameters are less pronounced. Nevertheless the tendency to the increase in juice and acid discharge at the stage of secretion is preserved.

The patients of Group 3 like in Group 1 the stimulating effect of HBO at the histamine stimulated stage of secretion is indisputable. In Group 4 with histamine resistant achlohydria the HBO therapy causes secretion changes.

The acceleration of the glandulocytes differentiation may account for the increase in free HCL level. The second major factor which promotes the restoration of gastric acid production might be the liquidation of regional hypoxy since the modern data shows that the process of HCL synthesis is strictly aerobic.

In patients with gastric and duodenal ulcer the HBO therapy leads to increase in gastric secretion which is not associated with major changes in gastrin concentrated in blood serum.

The increase in gastric secretion and free HCL discharge/hour on the background of quick ulcer healing under the HBO effect throws doubt on the importance of acido-peptic factor in the processes of ulcer formation and ulcer healing.

It was of great interest to study changes in free HCL discharge/hour under the influence of HBO in seccellular and cellular stimulus stimulation. To have a clear picture of the secretion changes the study was conducted in patients with chronic gastritis with hypochlorhydria. Histamine was used as a supcellular stimulus and theophylline as an intracellular.

At the basal stage of secretion free HCL production was not revealed. Histamine stimulation significantly decreased free HCL discharge/hour. After HBO therapy course (usually 10 sessions) discharge/hour increased in average up to 3m/hour/1. Using the combined stimulus histamine and theophylline significant increase of free HCL level was revealed. Therapeutic effect of HBO mainly at the stimulated stage of secretion in patients with chronic atrophic gastritis with hypochlorhydria (22 patients) was preserved for a long time of follow-up. (2 months - 2 years).

As any other type of ulcer treatment HBO method cannot be considered a universal one. First of all it should be kept in mind that the choice of patients for this treatment must be very careful. Since HBO enhances the proliferation processes we do not recommend this method if you suspect the malignant character of gastric ulcer. In 2 of 20 patients with chronic atrophic gastritis in two years after the treatment the formation of benign polyps was revealed. The interrelation of polyposis and HBO treatment needs further study.

Thus, the use of HBO in modern complex therapy of ulcers in the majority of cases leads to more rapid healing and increases the ulcer healing rate. HBO is the method of choice for gastric and duodenal ulcer persistent treatment. Still the mechanism of its effect is not clear completely. Probably, its positive effect is associated with several factors: 1) Regional hypoxia liquidation 2) Enhancement of adaptation-compensatory mechanisms. Among them the saturation of mucus with cellular elements, increased activity of mucus production and regenerating processes and also the redistribution of blood in arterial and venous systems of gastro-duodenal zone are of major importance.

Figure 1. Effect of HBO treatment on acetate ulcers healing in rats /model okabe/, 10 sessions, 14th day of the pathology, Morphometric analysis /mm/.

EFFECT OF HBO TREATMENT ON ACETATE STOMACH ULCERS HEALING IN RATS /MODEL OKABE/. 10 SESSIONS. 14-TH DAY OF THE PATHOLOGY. MORPHOMETRIC ANALYSIS /mm/

ACETATE STOMACH ULCER	CONTROL	EXPERIMENT	P
SIZE OF ULCERS	1.2±0.2	0.9±0.3	<0.05
THICKNESS OF NECROTIC MASS	0.14±0.002	0.06±0.003	<0.05
ZONE OF PHIBRINOUS NECROSIS	2.1±0.4	0.9±0.02	<0.05
EDGES EPITHELIZATION	1.2±0.3	2.04±0.07	<0.05
REGENERATING MUCOUSE MEMBRANE	0.3±0.01	1.2±0.04	<0.05

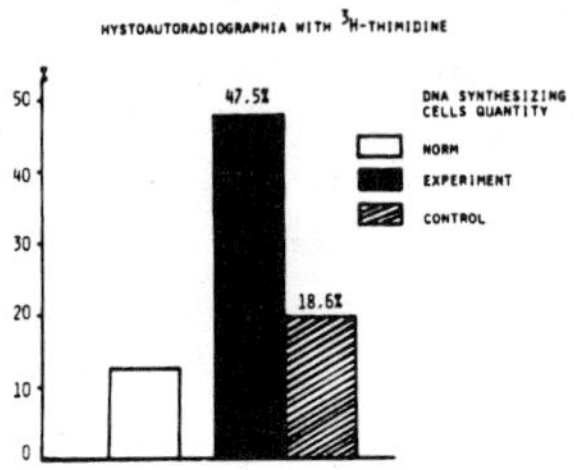

HYSTOAUTORADIOGRAPHIA WITH ^{3}H-THIMIDINE

DNA SYNTHESIZING CELLS QUANTITY
□ NORM
■ EXPERIMENT
▨ CONTROL

47.5% (EXPERIMENT), 18.6% (CONTROL)

COMPARATIVE EFFECT OF HBO AND VARIOUS AGENTS TREATMENT OF
PATIENTS WITH ULCER DESEASE

	TREATMENT EFFECT, %	AVERAGE PERIOD OF CICATRICE FORMATION /DAYS/
CARBENOXOLONE	71	36.5±1.3
ZOLLIMIDINE	65	35.5±3.8
SOLCOSERYLE	75	48.3±3.6
H$_2$-BLOCATERS /CIMETIDINE, TAGAMET/	87.5	27.0±3.6
H$_2$-BLOCATERS /RANITIDINE, ZANTAC/	84	28.2±2.9
EGLONILE /SULPIRIDE/	60	36.0±2.9
ANTEPSINE /SUCRALFAT/	80	28.2±4.3
HBO	92.5	21.8±1.1

Figure 2. Comparative effect of HBO and various agents treatment of patients with ulcer disease.

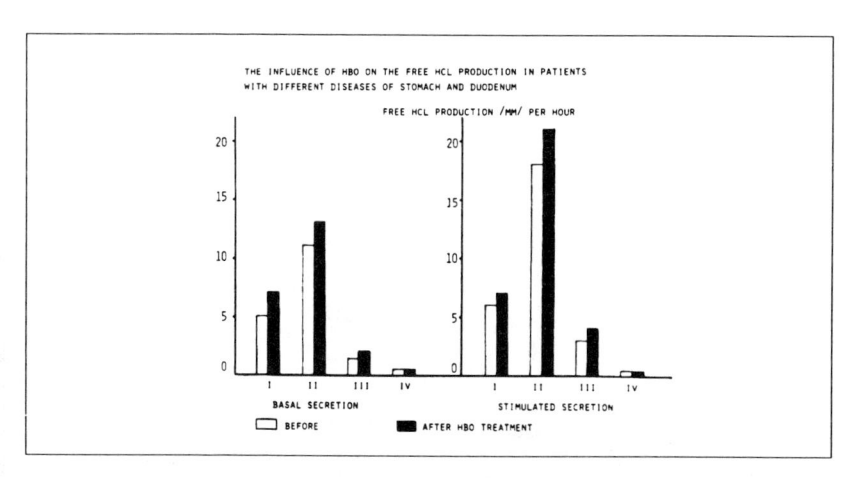

Figure 3. The influence of HBO on the free HCL production in patients with different diseases of stomach and duodenum.

Hyperbaric oxygen at 2.0 or 2.5 ATA as an adjunct to levodopa therapy of retinitis pigmentosa

A controlled study

A. Marroni, De Iuliis G. *, Di Marzio L., De Sanctis G., Modugno G.** and Data P. G. ***

Centro Iperbarico Polivente di Ricerca, S. Atto, Teramo, Italy
* Dept. of Ophtalmology, City Hospital, Teramo, Italy
** Dept. of Ophtalmology, Sapienza University, Rome, Italy
*** Dept. of Physiology, University of Chieti, Chieti, Italy

ABSTRACT

Retinitis Pigmentosa is a slowly progressing, hereditary, generally bacterial retinal degenerative disease of unknown ethiology for which local hypoxia seems to play an important role. Drugs so far used for the treatment of this condition have been of little use with the exception of Levodopa treatment which seems to slow down the evolution of the disease. 29 patients (average age 43.5 yrs, ave. disease duration 23 yrs) were randomly divided into 6 study groups. Group A1: Levodopa 125 + 12 mg/day + HBO at 2.0 ATA for 20 initial sessions of 90 min followed by 5 similar booster sessions every fifth week. Group A2: HBO at 2.0 ATA as above, no Levodopa. Group B1: HBO as above at 2.5 ATA + Levodopa. Group B2: HBO as above at 2.5 ATA, no Levodopa. Group C1: Levodopa only Group, no HBO. Group C2: control group, no treatment. Patients were evaluated for Perimetry, Visual Acuity, ERG and Patient Self Evaluation before entering the study, after the initial treatment sessions, then at three months after start. No variations were observed for ERG while a slight trend towards improvement of visual acuity was present in B1 group. Perimetry showed a well defined improvement in all HBO groups and best results were obtained at 2.0 ATA where an HBO effect could be seen independently from Levodopa. At 2.5 ATA the differential improvement was of lesser entity.

Patient Self Evaluation closely resembled the objective data. Observed improvements kept constant or furtherly increased with time. Levodopa-only Group showed same degree of differential improvement as the two 2.5 ATA Groups, while Control Group was the only one to show a worsening.

Key Words: HBO Therapy, Retinal Disease, Perimetry, ERG, Visual Acuity.

INTRODUCTION

Retinitis Pigmentosa is a slowly progressing, hereditary, generally bilateral retinal degenerative disease of unknown etiology (1).

It is thought (2) that in this disease the debris which accumulates on the external portion of the retinal rods, mainly lipidic in nature, may form a diffusion barrier between neural retina, pigment epithelium and choroidal circulation.

It was shown (2) that the time to blackout in normal human subjects following an increase in intraocular pressure to levels above arterial supply is a function of blood oxygenation.

Prebreathing 100% Oxygen markedly increases the time to blackout and decrease the time to complete functional recovery.

Retinitis Pigmentosa patients, on the other hand, do not show as clear an increase of the time to blackout and this was interpreted (2) as a sign of increased metabolic demand or smaller oxygen reservoir in these patients, possibly coupled with a diffusion barrier such as the debris on the rods outer segment between the choroidal circulation and the neural retina. It is also possible that the accumulated detached rod outer discs are still functional (2) and oxygen starved, thus imposing further demand on the oxygen diffusion at the expense of the photoreceptor retinal layer.

Hyperbaric Oxygen Therapy was used for this disease by some Researchers who reported promising results (3,4), but a certain debate exists about the optimal treatment pressure, some Authors (4) favoring pressures of 2.5-2.8 ATA, others (3) preferring lower pressures in consideration of the known circulatory and toxic effects of HBO on the eye (5,6,7) and the recently reported development of nuclear cataracts in long term HBO patients treated for ulcer healing or other soft tissue disorders (8).

The panoply of drugs for the disease is very little and the only one that seems now to yield some favorable results of stabilization or improvement is a Levodopa and Carbidopa combination (SINEMET r - 125+12 mg twice daily) (9).

We therefore decided to develop a controlled study protocol to investigate on the suitability of HBO therapy, as an adjunct to Levodopa or per se, as a treatment for Retinitis Pigmentosa.

MATERIALS AND METHODS

29 patients suffering from Retinitis Pigmentosa were selected for the study after obtaining informed consent. No difference was made amongst the usually accepted four types of hereditary transmission of the disease (10) while all patients were at Stage II or III of the disease according to the classification reported by Cavallacci (9). Changes in Visual Field were computed by measuring the percent variations of the functioning residual area, Visual Acuity - photopic - was computed in tenths, ERG was given the following

values: normality = 1; slight electrical reduction = 2; frank electric reduction = 3; absence of electric signal = 4.

All the ophtalmological tests were performed by the two specialists of our team in a single blind fashion, the specialist not knowing the group the patients belonged to nor any previous result. The tests were performed before the beginning of the study, then after 30 and 120 days.

At the same times the patients were asked to state whether they felt that they had improved, remained unvaried, or worsened.

The patients were randomly assigned to 6 study groups as follows:
Group A1: HBO at 2.0 ATA for 90 min. for a first cycle of 20 sessions (five days per week) followed by 5 similar booster sessions every fifth week, plus Levodopa & Carbidopa 125+12 mg (Sinemet r) twice per day after meals for the entire period of the study.
{n.3, age 41+-4, disease age 19+-9 yrs.}
Group A2: HBO at 2.0 ATA as above, no Sinemet
{n.7, age 47+-13, disease age 28+-11 yrs.}
Group B1: HBO at 2.5 ATA as above plus Sinemet
{n.5, age 42+-9, disease age 25+-7 yrs.}
Group B2: HBO at 2.5 ATA as above, no Sinemet
{n.4, age 44+-7, disease age 27+-10 yrs}
Group C1: only Sinemet as above, no HBO
{n.5, age 44+-8, disease age 15+-7 yrs.}
Group C2: control group, no treatment
{n.5, age 41+-6, disease age 22+-8 yrs}

At the end of the study the data were collected, mediated group by group and test by test and confronted with the values observed before starting. The data are reported in table 1.

Data regarding Visual Field (Perimetry) were again elaborated and the differential values at the last test were plotted against the starting values made equal to zero (fig. 1)

RESULTS

All the study groups but group C2 - the control one - showed some improvement in Perimetry; 1 patient of group C2 actually showed a slight reduction in the Visual Field, thus lowering the median value, while the other four didn't show any variation. The other two parameters - i.e. Visual Acuity and ERG - didn't show any significant variation, even if there was a 0.2/10ths average improvement in Group B1 patients and a -0.2/10ths average reduction in Group C2.

Subjective evaluation by patients showed that 70% approximately - see table 1, Groups A1 and A2 - of the patients treated with 2.0 ATA HBO declared that they had improved, were very happy with the treatment and thought it had improved their quality of life; the remaining part declared no variation had occurred, while non worsened.

Group B patients - HBO at 2.5 ATA - showed a different attitude, 60% of group B1 (HBO and Sinemet) declared they had improved, while only 25% of group B2 patients (HBO and no Sinemet) observed an improvement. The remaining parts declared no variations and none worsened.

Group C1 patients - Sinemet and no HBO - declared improvement by 40% and no variation by 60% and Group C2 patients - control group - declared no variation by 80% and a worsening by 20% (1 out of 5).

Average differential improvement in Visual Field (fig. 1) was very evident (+8%) for groups A1 and A2, less significant for groups B2, C1 and B1 (+4% and +3% respectively) and negative for group C2 (-1%).

DISCUSSION

Retinitis Pigmentosa is a long term progressing disease and short term studies are certainly not the best. We are actually planning to continue with the study for at least 2 years with the same group of patients, even if some difficulties start arising in keeping the control group patients out of any form of treatment as news circulate among patients and as it is day by day more difficult to withdraw, even out of justified scientific reasons, a form of treatment that appears to offer some improvement or at the very least a halting of the progression of an otherwise very pitiless disease.

We think that, even at this early point, some interesting considerations can be made on the basis of the data obtained by this study.

HBO treatment, as hereby described, seems to yield interesting results and widening of the visual fields of Retinitis Pigmentosa patients as well as Sinemet drug therapy. Actually drug treatment alone or associated with HBO treatment at 2.5 ATA produced identical average widening of visual field in our study.

Group B1 - HBO at 2.5 ATA and Sinemet - was the only one where a certain improvement of visual acuity was registered.

On the other hand, HBO at 2.5 ATA alone also produced an improvement in Perimetry, although of lesser entity, and subjective evaluation was less satisfactory in this group.

HBO at 2.0 ATA, alone or associated with Sinemet drug treatment produced identical and well defined improvement of Perimetry and an equally comparable positive subjective evaluation by patients.

It may be inferred that HBO at 2.0 ATA, given according to the protocol here described, per se and in association with Sinemet therapy, produces better results than Sinemet and/or HBO treatment at 2.5 ATA for the treatment of Retinitis Pigmentosa, probably out of a better balance between oxygen induced retinal demand. The reciprocal roles of HBO and Levodopa-Carbidopa are still to be defined.

Table 1

N. 29: males 17, females 12.
Ave. Age 43.5 yrs. +-13//Ave. disease duration 23 years +-10

group	test type	test 1 x	test 1 sd	test 2 x	test 2 sd	test 3 x	test 3 sd	subjective evaluation criterium	n.	%
A1	Perimetry %	18	15	21	16	26	19	improved	2	67
	Vis. Ac. 1/10	3	2	=	=	3	2	unvaried	1	33
	ERG	3.5	0.5	=	-	3.5	0.5	worsened	0	0
A2	Perimetry %	12	4	14	6	20	8	improved	5	71
	Vis. Ac. 1/10	0.3	0.2	=	=	0.3	0.2	unvaried	2	29
	ERG	3.5	0.5	=	=	3.5	0.5	worsened	0	0
B1	Perimetry %	8	2	9	2	11	3	improved	3	60
	Vis. Ac. 1/10	2.1	2	=	=	2.3	2	unvaried	2	29
	ERG	3.5	0.5	=	=	3.5	0.5	worsened	0	0
B2	Perimetry %	18	2	18	2	22	2	improved	1	25
	Vis. Ac. 1/10	2.6	2	=	=	2.6	2	unvaried	2	40
	ERG	3.5	0.5	=	=	3.5	0.5	worsened	0	0
C1	Perimetry %	14	8	=	=	18	9	improved	2	40
	Vis. Ac. 1/10	2.2	1.5	=	=	2.2	1.5	unvaried	3	60
	ERG	3.5	0.5	=	=	3.5	0.5	worsened	0	0
C2	Perimetry %	13	7	=	=	12	8	improved	0	0
	Vis. Ac. 1.10	2.3	2	=	=	2.1	2	unvaried	4	80
	ERG	3.5	0.5	=	=	3.5	0.5	worsened	1	20

Values of useful residual area of Visual Field (Perimetry %), Visual Acuity expressed in tenths (photopic), Electroretinogram (see text) and subjective evaluation of the different study groups at the tests performed before entering the protocol (test 1) and at day 30 and 120 after starting (tests 2 and 3). Subjective evaluations here reported refer to the data collected on test 3.

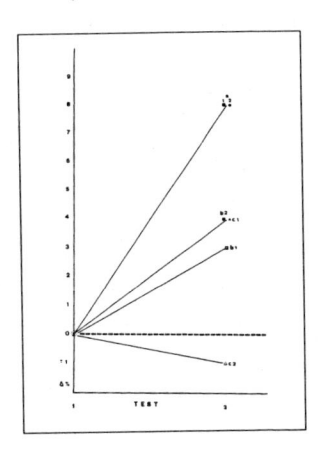

Figure 1. Mean differential variations of residual functioning visual field area in the different study groups.
A1: HBO 2.0 ATA and sinemet r, A2: HBO 2.0 ATA
B1: HBO 2.5 ATA and sinemet r, B2: HBO 2.5 ATA
C1: Sinemet r, C2: Control

REFERENCES

1. Cavallacci G, Marconcini A, Oliva A, Perossini M, Formaro P Nuovi orientamenti terapeurici della retinite pigmentosa alla luce di recenti acquisizioni di fisiologia retinica Proceeding of LX Congress of the Italian Ophtalmological Society: 211-223; 1980. Rome Italy
2. Wolbarsht ML, Landers MB, Wadsworth JAC, Anderson WB Retinitis Pigmentosa: Clinical Management and Current Concepts A Duke University Eye Center Report. Durham N.C. 1983
3. Modugno GC, Pelaia P, Palombi L OTI in alcune affezioniz di interesse oftalmologico Proceedings of the VIII SOS Congress, Taormina Italy 1983
4. Oriano G, Musini A, Barnini C, Pedesini C, Gaietta T Su un protocollo di terapia con ossigeno iperbarico nel trattamento della retinite pigmentosa Med. Sub. Iper. 4(3): 7-14; 1984
5. Lambertsen CJ Effect of Hyperoxia on Organs and their Tissues In: Extrapulmonary Manifestations of Respiratory Disease E.D. Robin Ed. Lung Biology in Health and Disease Vol. 8: 239-303; 1978
6. Nichols CW, Lambertsen CJ Effects of Oxygen upon Ophtalmic Structures In: Underwater Physiology: 57-66; 1969 CJ Lambertsen Ed. Academic Press, New York
7. Nicholos CW, Yanoff M, Hall DA, Lambertsen CJ Histologic Alteration Produced in the Eye by Oxygen at High Pressure Arch. Ophtalm. 87: 417-421; 1972
8. Palmquist BM, Philipson B, Olof Barr P Nuclear Cataract and Myopia during Hyperbaric Oxygen Therapy Brit. J. Ophtal. 68: 113-117; 1984 9. Cavallacci G, Genovesi Ebert A, Mannini C, Marconcini C, Oliva A, Pucci G
9. Le basi teoriche ed i risultati cliniici della terapia con L-Dopa Proceedings of the LXII Congress of the Italian Ophtalmological Society: Rome Italy; 1982
10. Pearlman JT, Mathematical Models of Retinitis Pigmentosa: a Study of the Rate of Progress in the Different Genetic Forms Tr. Am. Ophtal. Soc. 77: 643; 1979.

Studies involving animal experiments to identify the action of hyperbaric oxygen on the inner ear

Pilgramm M, Mann W, Lohle E, Fischer B[*], Frey G[**],
Lamm K[***] and Schmutz J[****]

ENT University Hospitald Freiburg
West Germany (Director: Prof. Dr. Chl. Beck)
[*]Fachklinik der LVA Klausenbach
West Germany (Director: Prof. Dr. B. Fischer)
[**]Department X, Anaesthesia and Intensive Medicine
Federal German Army Hospital Ulm
West Germany (Senior Physician: P.D. Dr. E. Lenhardt)
[***]Department ENT, Hanover Medical School,
West Germany (Director: Prof. Dr. E. Lenhardt
[****]Foundation for Hyperbaric Medicine
Basle, Switzerland (Director: Dr. J. Schmutz)

Author's address: M. Pilgramm M.D., Abteilung V, HNO, Bundeswehrkrankenhaus Ulm, Oberer Eselsberg 40, 7900 Ulm, West Germany

ABSTRACT

The clinical results obtained over the past few years in conjunction with the application of hyperbaric oxygen therapy to patients suffering acute inner ear damage prompted us to carry out investigations to establish at which point of the inner ear the hyperbaric oxygen acts. Two of these studies involving animal experiments are presented below.

1. Problem:
Does hyperbaric oxygenation cause an increase in the partial pressure of oxygen in the lymph in the inner ear?

2. Problem:
Does hyperbaric oxygen influence the histological picture of inner ear sensory cells that have been damaged through acoustic trauma?
Our findings were the following:

Through the hyperbaric oxygenation that we selected, it is possible to achieve a six-fold increase in the partial pressure of oxygen in the lymph that supplies the inner ear sensory cell.

If hyperbaric oxygenation therapy is commenced in time, the acoustic damage to the inner ear can be largely prevented or reserved.

In a number of clinical studies conducted on a strictly randomized basis, we have been able to show over the past few years that, in the case of acute acoustic trauma and sudden deafness, hyperbaric oxygenation combined with a standard therapy is superior to the standard therapy in isolation at a statistically significant level.

With patients suffering from sudden deafness, the average hearing gain in patients treated with hyperbaric oxygen is some 10 dB greater than in patients treated with the standard therapy. Hyperbaric oxygenation is similarly far superior for the control of tinnitus.

The same applies to an even greater extent with acute acoustic trauma. Here, a hearing gain that is 16 dB higher on average can be achieved, and whilst only one patient with acoustic trauma damage reported no more tinnitus following the standard therapy, the figure for the hyperbaric group was 3.5 patients.

These results greatly encouraged us, particularly since they stood up to all the statistical tests. We thus set ourselves the target of reconstructing our clinical studies in animal experiments.

Two of these studies involving animal experiments are present below:

STUDIES

1. We investigated whether it was possible to achieve an increase in the partial pressure of oxygen inside the lymph by means of hyperbaric oxygenation, since it is from these fluids that the inner ear sensory cell receives it principal nourishment.

2. We looked into whether hyperbaric oxygenation has an influence on the histological picture of inner ear sensory cells that have been damaged by acoustic trauma.

ON STUDY 1:

Figure 1 shows that test setup for measuring the oxygen in the inner ear. We used a measuring probe which operates on a polarographic basis. This was introduced into the inner ear via the round window by means of a nanostepper. The probe has a tip diameter of roughly 1 mm and was constructed under the direction of a working party at the Max Planck Institute in Dortmund, West Germany (Prof. Lubbers, Dr. Baumgartl).

The guinea pigs used for the experiments (n=30) were all white, female, 250 to 300g in weight and had a clearly obtainable Preyer's reflex of the outer ear.

The anaesthesia used was an injection anaesthesia with a combination of 15 ml Rompun^R (1mg Xylazin per 100g body weight) and 60 ml Ketanest^R (11 mg Ketaminbase per 100g body weight), applied in. After preparation had been completed a further 25ml Ketanest was injected ip.

Whilst the ear was being prepared and later, during the measurement procedure proper, the animal lay on a heated operating table with a head rest, which stood on the base of the hyperbaric chamber. In the course of preparation, the right ear was removed, after shaving, and the bulla carefully opened from the post-occipital direction using small bone forceps under microscopic control. Sufficient bony tissue had to be removed for the round window membrane to be clearly visible and readily accessible. Bipolator coagulation forceps were used to control hemorrhage. The application of drops of hot wax, again with the bipolator forceps, successfully prevented any tissue lymph from seeping out of the surrounding area. It was then possible to move the electrode close enough to the round window membrane at the correct angle of puncture (approximately 45 degree) under microscopic control for the chamber bell to be safely clapped over. The probe was then inserted using an electrically adjustable nanostepper with facilities for infinitely variable or stepped adjustment in the X-Y-Z direction; this had the electrode clamped into its holder.

After the chamber had been closed, the tip of the probe was inserted 100 to 200mm into the round window membrane by means of the nanostepper until a steady, uniform measuring signal was obtained following the initial unsteadiness and fluctuations. The tip of the probe was then advanced to a penetration depth of 1200mm in 100mm steps at two minute intervals. The chamber was then rinsed with medical oxygen for ten minutes in order to produce a pure oxygen environment. A fifteen-minute chamber run (hyperbaric oxygen) was then commenced up to 1.5 bar overpressure, with a pressure buildup of 0.1 bar/min. After four minutes' constant overpressure of 1.5 bar, the probe was withdrawn again as far as the membrane, on a step by step basis - in the same way as it had been introduced.

Figure 2 shows the reduction current curve during an animal experiment. The ordinate gives the reduction current flow nanoamperes and the abscissa the path travelled by the probe into the inner ear.

If the current curves of 30 animals are evaluated, the following results are obtained.

Rinsing with oxygen produces a current increase of 267 ± 129%.

Flooding the chamber to 1.5 bar overpressure gives a current increase of 649 ± 214%.

What is interesting here is the fact that relatively constant values are obtained for the O_2 increase through the chamber being rinsed with O_2. The O_2 measurements under hyperbaric conditions in the inner ear, however, reveal greater differences, even though a detailed check was made on individual probes prior to each measurement.

We can thus say that not all animals react to hyperbaric therapy with an equally high level of oxygen enrichment in the lymph.

From these results it can be concluded at the same time that the hyperbaric oxygen treatment produces an increase in the partial pressure of oxygen in the lymph, firstly through direct diffusion through the two window membranes and secondly through increased deoxygenaton of the vessels supplying the inner ear.

We have learned from this experiment that we can be certain that hyperbaric oxygenation produces increased oxygen tension in the inner ear sensory cell and that it is possible to compensate the oxygen deficit brought about by acoustic overloading.

ON STUDY 2:

We exposed guinea pigs (n=30) that were 15 to 18 weeks old and weighed between 250 and 300g to the same acoustic trauma frequently experienced by soldiers in the armed forces in West Germany. Six shots were fired within one minute from the same small firearm (G3 Federal Army gun) at a distance of 25 to 30cm from the each conch. This gives a sound peak of some 156 dB at the ear-drum.

The guinea pigs then either remained untreated or received hyperbaric therapy in an animal chamber.

THERAPEUTIC SCHEME:

Ten ten-minute sessions of oxygen therapy within 60 hours with 100% oxygen at 1.5 bar overpressure. Therapy to commence four hours after the acoustic trauma event.

Sixty hours after the acoustic trauma event, the inner ears of all the animals were removed and dissected, and the inner ear sensory cells in the region of the transition from the first to the second spiral canal of the cochlea were counted using an interference contrast microscope. These findings were compared with a standard animal group.

If the morphologically healthy cells in the three groups are counted under the interference contrast phase microscope taking 20 ears in each group and about 20000 cells, then the following result is obtained:

Taking a count range of 31.25mm, it is possible to count 8.9 healthy outer hair cells for the control group, 6.0 for the group exposed to shooting and 7.6 healthy outer hair cells for the group that was exposed to shooting and received oxygen treatment.

With the same count range of 31.25mm, it is possible to count 3.2 healthy inner hair cells in the control group, 2.4 in the group exposed to shooting and 2.6 healthy inner hair cells in the group that was exposed to shooting and received oxygen treatment.

The lower figures for the inner hair cells compared with the outer hair cells are explained by the fact that there are three rows of out hair cells and only one row on inner hair cells.

As far as significance is concerned, the differences between all three groups are highly significant in the case of the outer hair cells ($p<0.001$).

In the case of the inner hair cells, there is a high level of significance ($p<0.05$) between the other two pairs of groups.

The statistically significant results of this test series showed us that if hyperbaric oxygenation is applied in time following acute acoustic trauma then it is possible to either prevent or reverse a large part of the damage to the inner ear.

Through our animal experiments we were additionally able to show that:

1. Through the hyperbaric oxygenation we selected, it is possible to increase the oxygen content of the lymph that supplies the inner ear sensory cell and that

2. by commencing oxygenation therapy in time, acoustic damage to the inner ear can be largely prevented or reversed.

We are aware of the fact that many work groups have doubted our clinical results and thus shied away from giving hyperbaric treatment to inner ear patients. We are thus letting the clinical studies run further and soon hope to be able to confirm the results we have achieved in previous years on much larger groups of patients precisely since the results of our animal experiments have underlined our clinical finding.

Figure 1. Hyperbaric chamber and test setup

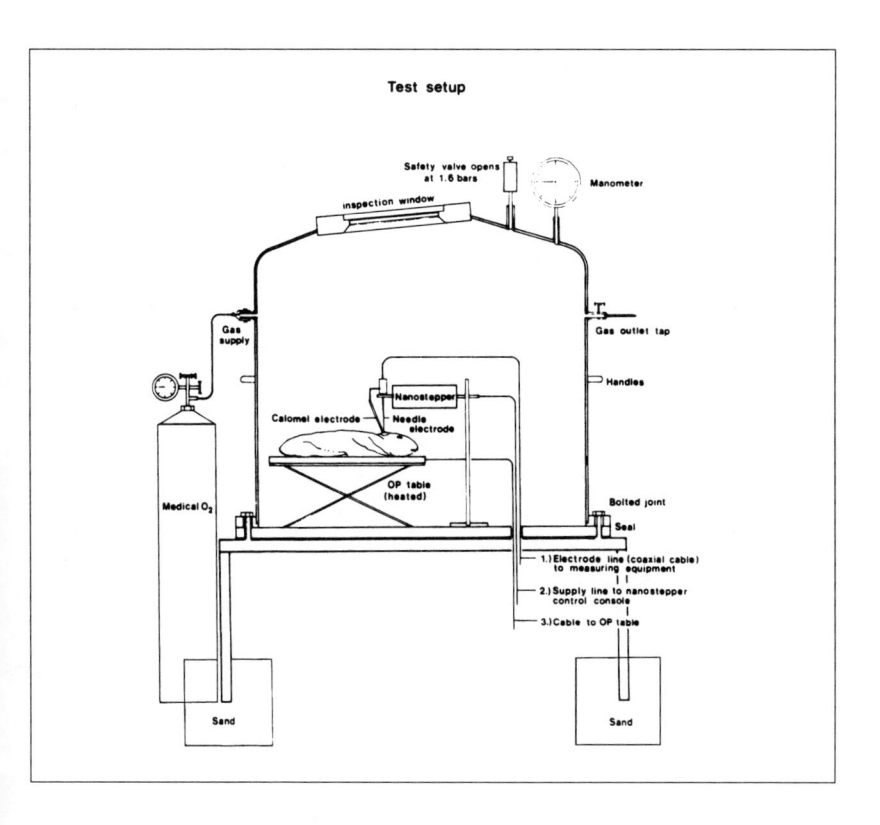

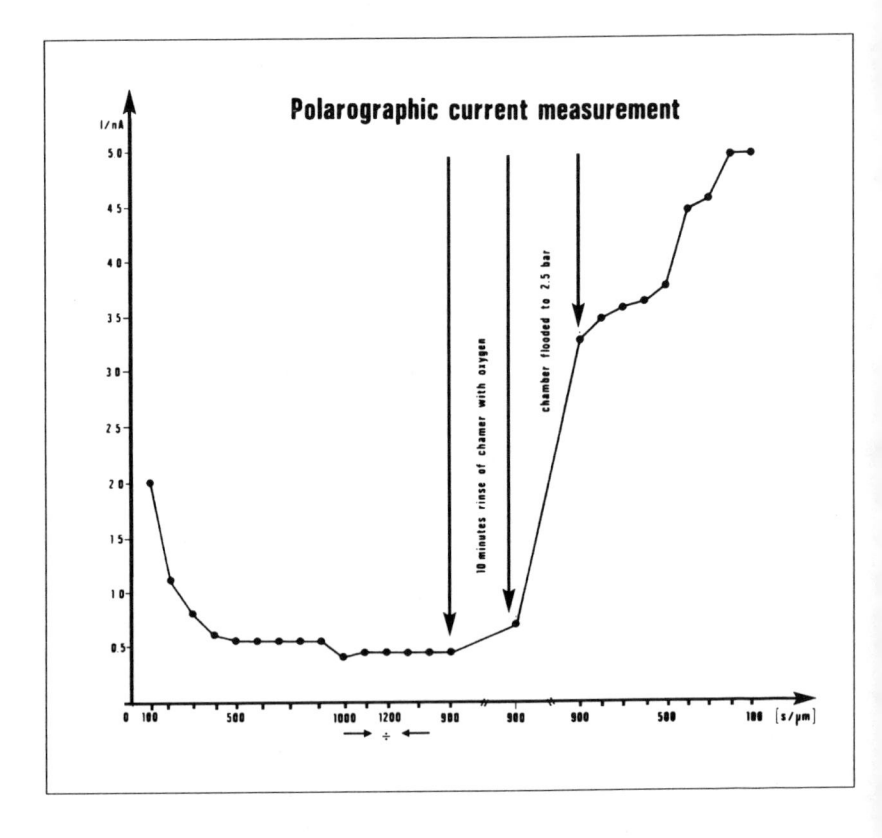

Figure 2. Change in current flow (proportional to the change in O_2 concentration) during a measurement in the lymph of the inner ear of a guinea pig.

Hyperbaric oxygen therapy in recent spinal cord injury

John D. Yeo, A.O., M.B., M.S., D.P.R.M., F.R.A.C.S., F.A.C.R.M.

Spinal Injuries Unit,
Royal North Shore Hospital
Sydney, Australia

SUMMARY

Fifty two patients with spinal cord lesions have been treated with hyperbaric oxygen (HBO). Patients were given one, two or three treatments, usually 90 minutes induration at 2.5 atmospheres absolute.

Of the 52 patients with spinal cord injury, 45 patients had upper motor neurone lesions. Thirty-four patients in this group had two or three pressurization (2.5ATA). Of these, 15 had significant functional recovery (44%) and 19 little or no significant recovery (56%). The remaining eight patients had only one period of pressurization with no identifiable response to treatment. The average delay in commencing HBO after the spinal cord injury was nine hours.

All patients with useful recovery had some clinical evidence of spinal cord function below the level before treatment.

INTRODUCTION

Previous studies on spinal cord injury indicate ischaemia plays a significant role in the permanent loss of neuronal function following trauma to the spinal cord. (C.N.S. Trauma, 1984 Vol. 1, No. 2 p. 161-165).

This study reviews that effects of hyperbaric oxygen (HBO) on patients with recent spinal cord injury admitted within hours to the specialized Spinal Injuries Unit (40 beds) situated within a 900 bed University teaching hospital.

MATERIALS AND METHODS

Fifty-two patients with spinal cord injury received hyperbaric oxygen therapy.

Forty-five patients with upper motor neurone lesions of the spinal cord received one, two or three pressurizations, 90 minutes in duration at 2.5 atmospheres absolute. The patients tolerance to the 90 minutes of pressurization determined the number of treatment given and eight patients who had only one treatment were excluded from the clinical study.

Thirty-four patients had two or three pressurizations commencing within 14 hours after injury. Twenty-seven patients had cervical lesions and seven had thoracic lesions.

Treatments were given in a Vickers single place, closed circuit unit, with console. The average delay in commencing hyperbaric oxygen after injury was nine hours. (Range 4-14 hours).

Recovery of motor power and sensation below the level of the lesion (54 patients). Grade A: Complete loss of motor and sensory function. Grade B: Some sensation present. Grade C: Some motor power present. Grade D: Useful motor power. Grade E: Normal.

* SCALE FOR MUSCLE STRENGTH EVALUATION

0 = muscle incapable of any contraction
1 = flicker
2 = joint movement with gravity eliminated
3 = joint movement against gravity
4 = movement against gravity and slight resistance
5 = movement against gravity and increased resistance
6 = normal motor power and range of motion

Clinical examinations recording motor, sensory and reflex activity were reported on numerous occasions to assess progress. Patients were categorized into clinical groups at the time of admission, prior to treatment, and if indicated re-categorized into another clinical group before discharge from hospital. The period of hospitalization varied between three and five months.

CONTROLS:

Sixty-three patients with upper motor neurone lesions treated without hyperbaric oxygen were grouped into the above clinical categories on admission and prior to discharge. The treatment of these patients was similar in all other respects: 55 (85.5%) had cervical spinal cord injury and 8 (12.5%) had thoracic lesions.

Significant functional recovery was recorded in the patient who recovered through at least two clinical categories (i.e. A to C, B to D, C to E) prior to discharge.

Insignificant functional recovery was recorded when the patient had no recovery or improved through only one clinical category (i.e. A to B, B to C, C to D or D to E) prior to discharge.

RESULTS

In a randomized series of 63 patients who did not receive HBO treatment 29 (46%) had significant functional recovery before discharge. In the 34 HBO treated patients 15 (46%) had significant recovery.

In both the control and HBO treated groups all patients who had significant recovery had some evidence of spinal cord function below the level of the lesion before treatment commenced.

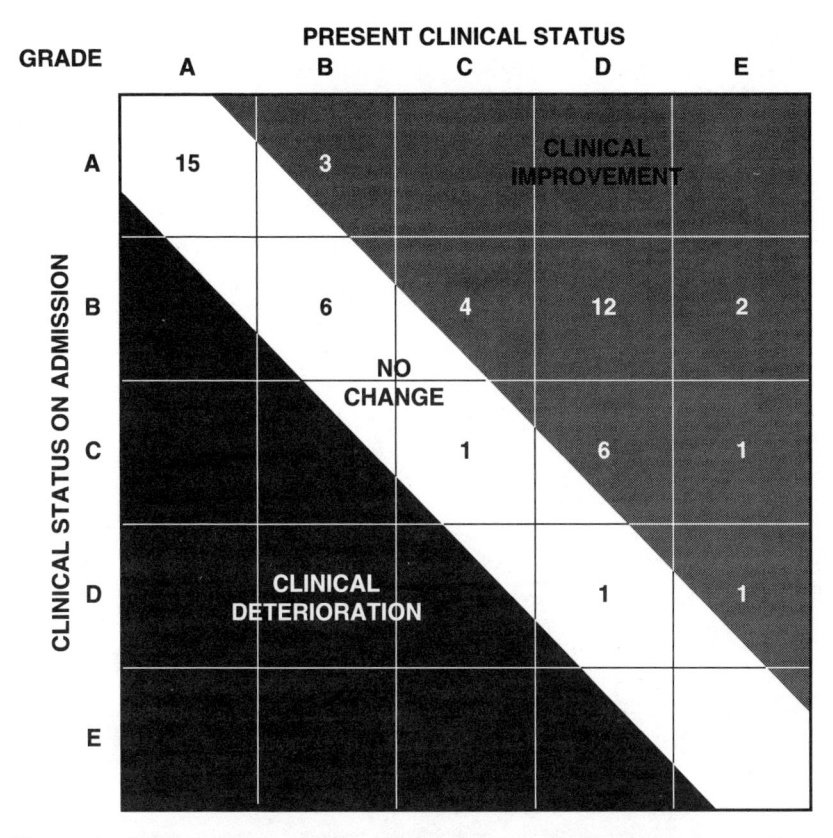

	A	B	C	D	E
A	15	3		CLINICAL IMPROVEMENT	
B		6	4	12	2
C			1	6	1
D		CLINICAL DETERIORATION		1	1
E					

GRADE (rows: CLINICAL STATUS ON ADMISSION; columns: PRESENT CLINICAL STATUS). Diagonal: NO CHANGE.

Figure 1. HBO treated patients. Recovery of motor power and sensation below the level of the lesion (54 patients). Grade A: Complete loss of motor & sensory function. Grade B: Some sensation present. Grade C: Some motor power present. Grade D: Useful motor power. Grade E: Normal.

DISCUSSION

It is important to acknowledge the impressive number of patients with functional recovery (46%) in the group who did not have hyperbaric oxygen treatment. The number of those with significant functional recovery following treatment in specialized spinal units is obviously increasing, suggesting improved techniques in first aid and the appropriate choice of transportation for early specialized treatment in the Spinal Unit.

Several years after the commencement of this study a report was published indicating that hyperbaric oxygen appeared to promote early recovery of motor power following spinal cord injury (Gamache, F.W., Myers, F.A.M., Ducker T.B.and Cowley, R.A. 1981). Although this preliminary report was encouraging, further work was necessary to prove whether the final degree of clinical recovery in the patient with an incomplete spinal cord lesion is greater when that patient has received hyperbaric oxygen treatment as an adjunct to standard medical procedures. Correction of the bony injury and stabilization of the vertebral canal are necessary to maximize recovery in all patients with an incomplete spinal cord lesion.

No patients with a clinically complete lesion appeared to benefit from hyperbaric oxygen in this series. Although the average delay in commencing treatment was 9 hours, several patients commenced HBO as late as 14 hours after injury and this delay may mitigate against the success of HBO therapy.

The depth of 2.5 atmospheres absolute was chosen to maximize the effects of oxygen diffusion in neural tissue but to avoid the increasing incidence of oxygen toxicity when higher pressures are used. No complications from HBO treatment were reported in this series (Hollin, S.A., Espinosa, O.E., Sukoff, M.H. and Jacobson II, J.H. 1968: Sukoff, 1978: Yeo, Lowry and McKenzie, 1978: Jones, Unsworth and Marosszeky, 1979).

Further research should continue in the use of hyperbaric oxygen therapy to protect the injured spinal cord from the effects of delayed ischaemia. Accurate assessment of the degree of injury to the spinal cord is fundamental to a satisfactory scientific evaluation of this treatment. Interpretation of the spinal cord injury from the clinical examination of the recently injured patient is difficult due to the physiological phenomenon of "spinal shock." Sensory evoked potentials will assist in defining the extent of injury to the spinal cord. (Higgins, Pearlstein, Mullen, Blaine and Mashold, 1981: Chehrazi, Wagner, Collins and Freeman, 1981: Linke, Holbach, Wassman and Hoheluchter, 1975).

It will be important in the future to identify those patients with some spared spinal cord function but who, for several days, appear clinically to have a "complete" spinal cord lesion. These patients could also experience motor and sensory recovery if the complicating post-traumatic ischaemia was modified.

ACKNOWLEDGEMENTS

I have been greatly assisted by my colleagues, Drs. Bart McKenzie and Cris J. Lowry, Consultant Anesthesiologist and Consultants in Hyperbaric Medicine.

SELECTED REFERENCES

1. Chehrazi, B., Wagner, F.C., Collins, W.F. and Freeman, D.H. 1981. A scale for evaluation of spinal cord injury. J. Neurosurg, 54, 310.
2. Gamache, F.W., Myers, R.A.M., Ducker, T.B. and Cooley, R.A. 1981. The clinical application of hyperbaric oxygen therapy in spinal cord injury: a preliminary report. Surgical Neurology, 15,85.
3. Hartzog, J.T., Fisher, R.G. and Snow, C. 1969. Spinal cord trauma effect of hyperbaric oxygen therapy. 17th S.C.I. conference. Veterans Administration published proceedings, 70.
4. Higgins, A.C., Pearlstein, R.D., Mullen, J.B., Nashold, B.S. 1981. Effects of hyperbaric oxygen therapy on long-tract neuronal conduction in the acute phase of spinal cord injury. J. Neurosurg, 55, 50.
5. Holbach, K.H., Wassman, H., and Linke, D. 1971. The use of hyperbaric oxygenation in the treatment of spinal cord lesions. Eur. Neurol, 16, 213.
6. Holbach, K.H., Wassman, H. Hoheluchter, K.L., Linke, D nad Ziemann, B. 1975. Cliniconeurological development of spinal lesions under hyperbaric oxygenation treatment HO Adv. Neurosurg., 2, 262.
7. Hollin, S.A., Espinosa, O.E., Sukoff, H.M. and Jacobsen, II, J.H. 1968, The effect of hyperbaric oxygenation on cerbrospinal fluid oxygen. J. Neurosurg., 29, 229.
8. Jones, R.F., Unsworth, I.P., and Marosszeky, J.E. 1978. Hyperbaric oxygen and acute spinal cord injuries in humans. Med. J. Aust., 2, 573.
9. Kelly, D.L., Jr., Lassiter, K.R.L., Vongsvivut, A. and Smith, J.M. 1972. Effects of hyperbaric oxygenation and tissue oxygen studies in experimental paraplegia. J. Neurosurg., 36, 425.
10. Linke, D., Holbach, K.H., Wassmann, H. and Hoheluchter, K.L. 1975. Electromyographic surveillance of hyperbaric oxygenation treatment of HO of spinal lesions. Adv. Neurosurg., 2, 268.
11. Maeda, N. (1965) Experimental studies on the effect of decompression procedures and hyperbaric oxygenation for the treatment of spinal cord injury. Nara Medical Assoc., 16, 429.
12. Sukoff, M.H. 1980. Central nervous system: review and update, cerebral oedema and spinal cord injuries. H.B.O. Review, 1, 189.
13. Yeo, J.D. 1977. A review of experimental research in spinal cord injury. Paraplegia, 14, 1.
14. Yeo, J.D., Stabback, S., McKenzie, B. 1977. Experimental: spinal cord injury: Proceeding 6th International Congress on Hyperbaric Medicine, 233, Aberdeen University Press, Scotland.
15. Yeo, J.D., Lowry, C. and McKenzie, B. 1978: Preliminary report on ten patients with spinal cord injuries treated with hyperbaric oxygen. Med. J. Aust. 2, 572.
16. Yeo, J.D., 1984. The use of Hyperbaric Oxygen to Modify the Effects of Recent Contusion Injury to the Spinal Cord.
17. Central Nervous System Trauma, Vol. 1, No.2, p.161-165.

The effect of pressure on the induction of ocular hyperuricosis

William J. Ehler, Charles H. Bonney*, Kwok-Wai Lam* and John H. Cissik

Clinical Investigation Facility,
Wilford Hall USAF Medical Centre,
Lackland AFB, Texas, USA 78236-5300
*Department of Ophthalmology,
University of Texas Health Science Center at
San Antonio, Texas, USA 78284

The opinions expressed herein are those of the authors and are not necessarily those of the United States Air Force or the Department of Defense.
(Supported by funds from the United States Air Force and by a grant from Research to Prevent Blindness)

ABSTRACT

Uric acid in the aqueous humor (ocular hyperuricosis) is an abnormal constituent. Patients exposed to hyperbaric oxygen (HBO) have been reported to have myopic changes in vision, and the development of cataracts. Ocular hyperuricosis, in experimental animals, has been induced both pharmacologically, and with exposure to HBO. From the results of the HBO study, the question was raised as to the effect of oxygen versus the effect of pressure on the biochemical composition of the eye. Changes in aqueous humor composition could explain the reported changes in vision.

In this study, New Zealand white rabbits were exposed to either ambient air (air divers) or 100% oxygen (HBO) at 2.4 ATA (45 feet of sea water of 13.72 meters) for periods of 90 minutes for a total of 60 dives. The control group of 12 animals was exposed to ambient air alone. The control group was found to have mean uric acid value of 0.12 mg/dl (+0.1) as compared to the treatment group averages of 0.35 mg/dl (air divers) and 0.32 mg/dl (HBO). The treatment means were significantly different ($P<0.001$) from the control mean. The results suggest that the induction of uric acid in aqueous humor is related to the increased pressure and not directly to the oxygen concentration.

INTRODUCTION

Following multiple exposures to hyperbaric oxygen (HBO), the eyes of many patients have been reported to develop myopia while others have developed myopia and nuclear cataracts (1,2). The myopia is an immediate response and is considered to be due to reversible changes in the lens. The nuclear cataract development is delayed (6 months to a year) phenomenon (1). Experimentally, exposure to HBO has produced changes in corneal endothelium in guinea-pigs (3), and lens epithelial changes in both guinea-pigs and mice (4).

The maintenance of the intraocular pressure and the nutrition of the cornea and lens is dependent upon the formation and composition of the fluid filling the anterior segment, the aqueous humor. In this study, aqueous humor samples taken from control rabbits, rabbits exposed to HBO, and rabbits exposed to hyperbaric air were analyzed for levels of uric acid.

METHODS AND MATERIALS

Adult, mixed sex New Zealand white rabbits ranging in weight from 2 to 3 kilograms were used in this study. Twelve rabbits were used in the control group and were exposed to ambient air only. Fifteen rabbits were used in the HBO treatment group and seventeen rabbits were used in the air diver treatment group.

The HBO treatment group of rabbits, in individual wire cages, were placed into a Rheem diving chamber. No medications were administered. The chamber was flushed with 100% oxygen until and oxygen concentration of 95-96% was reached. It took approximately 10 to 15 minutes to attain this concentration. When the final oxygen concentration was reached, the chamber pressure was increased to 2.4 ATA (45 feet of sea water of 13.72 meters). At this time the timing of the dive began. Oxygen concentration within the chamber was monitored with a Beckman oxygen analyzer. Carbon dioxide levels within the chamber were also monitored using a Beckman carbon dioxide analyzer. The relative humidity within the chamber was kept in the range of 35-60 percent. After a 90 minute exposure to HBO, the chamber was depressurized to 1 ATA in approximately 10 minutes. This procedure was repeated daily, five days a week, until a total of 60 dives had been conducted. No animals received more than one dive per day.

The air diver group followed an identical dive profile in the same Rheem chamber. While breathing ambient air, these animals were also compressed to 2.4 ATA (45 feet of sea water or 13.72 meters) for 90 minutes. The CO_2 levels were monitored with the Beckman CO_2 analyzer. The chamber was periodically flushed with air to maintain a relative humidity of 35-60 percent. This group likewise received a total of 60 dives.

Collection of aqueous humor samples was conducted in the following manner: anesthesia was induced with an intramuscular injection of ketamine (60mg/kg) and topical anesthetic was applied to the corneas (1% proparacaine). Samples were collected by paracentesis, under a Zeiss surgical microscope at 25 x, using a 30 gauge needle attached to a 1 milliliter syringe. Aqueous humor was taken from each eye, immediately placed on ice, and maintained separately for analysis. Thus, the statistical analysis of the control group was based on 24 samples, the HBO treatment group on 30 samples, and the air diver group on 34 samples.

The aqueous humor was analyzed for uric acid using high performance liquid chromatography (HPLC). The column was a microbondapak-NH_2 column (Waters Associates) designed for the separation of biochemical constituents in aqueous humor. The column was equilibrated in 10mM NH_4 $H_2 PO_4$ and eluted with the same buffer.

RESULTS

None of the animals were found to have lens opacities as viewed at the time of aqueous humor sample collection.

The mean uric acid level for the control group was 0.12 mg/dl (± .103), 0.32 mg/dl (±.19 (for the HBO treatment group, and 0.35 mg/dl (±0.1) for the air diver group. The control and treatment group means were analyzed using the two-tailed t-test. The mean uric acid levels were found to be significantly different (P<0.001) for both the air diver and the HBO groups vs the control group concurrently. See Table 1. There was no significant difference between the treatment means (P>0.05).

DISCUSSION

This study was designed to compare ocular uric acid levels in HBO and air divers. The study was not designed to look for nuclear cataracts. HBO exposures, as used in this study, might show such changes if the animals were held for a number of months.

In man, the uric acid is the final metabolic product of the metabolism of the purines, adenine and guanine. These compounds may be found within cells linked to deoxyribose-5-phosphate, forming two of the four basic units of chromosomal DNA, and they combine with ribose-5-phosphate to form two of the structural units of RNA. Hormonal effects are mediated by cyclic AMP which also contains these purines. Purines may be liberated by enzymatic degradation of tissue (5).

Normally, aqueous humor contains only trace amounts of uric acid (6). The initial report of significant levels of uric acid in aqueous humor was from eyes with glaucoma that had been treated medically for years prior to the surgery (7). The questions raised by the discovery of uric acid in aqueous humor addressed the source of uric acid, and its role in either the physiology of the eye or the pathology of glaucoma. In an experimental model of hyperuricemia, Yonentani found evidence that production of uric acid was associated with stimulation of alpha adrenergic receptors by the systematic administration of epinepherine (8). Similar data for alpha receptors in the eye does not exist. The source of intraocular uric acid has been addressed in two experimental studies. No significant elevation of uric acid was found (9). A second study evaluated epinepherine topically applied to the cornea of rabbits (10). The rabbit aqueous humor samples were found to have a significant elevation of uric acid. These studies indicate a blood-aqueous barrier to uric acid, and that the uric acid arises from reactions within the eye.

Uric acid within eyes of rabbits treated with HBO and air diver is a new finding. Aqueous humor samples taken several hours following the last dive showed uric acid levels significantly elevated compared to the control samples. The fact that there was not a significant difference between the air diver and HBO experimental group uric acid means, however, indicates that the induction of uric acid in aqueous humor is related to the increase in total pressure rather than to the oxygen concentration.

The mean experimental values reported in this study, on the other hand, may actually represent figures lower than truly produced. This could be the result of either enzymatic activity of uricase, an enzyme not found in man, or from intraocular turnover. Washout of the uric acid by the constant formation and outflow of aqueous humor would produce a decay of the uric acid unless it was being added to the aqueous humor on a continual basis.

In the case of HBO, it is not known if the appearance of uric acid is related to the increase in tissue oxygenation, or to a regional ischemia secondary to the oxygen vasoconstrictive effects on blood vessels and resulting decreased perfusion (11). Nor is it yet known if the production of uric acid is from alter biochemistry or from cell death. If it is the former, it is suspected that it would be a transient event but with perhaps permanent ocular tissue changes.

In neither the pharmacologically produced nor the HBO-pressure produced ocular hyperuricosis is the presence of uric acid understood in terms of ocular physiology. The known changes, myopia and nuclear cataracts, may be related to changes in the composition of the aqueous humor.

"The experiments reported herein were conducted according to the principles set forth in National Institutes of Health (NIH) Publication No. 85-23, "Guide for the Care and Use of Laboratory Animals."

Table 1. Mean Urid Acid Levels in Rabbit Aqueous Humor.

	n	$\bar{x}$	SEM
Control Group:			
Uric Acid	24	0.012 mg/dl	0.02
HBO Diver Group:			
Uric Acid	30	0.32 mg/dl	0.06
Air Diver Group:			
Uric Acid	34	0.35 mg/dl	0.06

REFERENCES

1. Palmquist B-M, Philipson B, Barr P-O: Nuclear cataract and myopia during hyperbaric oxygen therapy. Brit J Ophthal 68: 113-117, 1984
2. Lyne AJ: Ocular effects of hyperbaric oxygen. Trans Ophthal Soc U K 98: 66-68, 1978.
3. Nichols CW, Yanoff M, Hall DA, Lambertsen CJ: Histologic alterations produced in the eye by oxygen at high pressure. Arch Ophthal 87: 417-421, 1972.
4. Schocket SS, Esterson J, Bradford B, Michaelis M, Richards RD: Induction of cataracts in mice by exposure to oxygen. Israel J Med Sci 8: 1596-1603, 1972.
5. Sorensen LB: A primer on purine metabolism. In: Gout: A clinical comprehensive, pp 20-24. Mecom Learning Systems, Burroughs Wellcome Co., Research Triangle Park, North Carolina 27709, 1971.
6. Gaasterland De, Pederson JE, MacLellan HM < Reddy VN: Rhesus monkey aqueous humor composition and a primate ocular perfusate. invest Ophthal Vis Sci 18: 1139 - 1150, 19769.
7. Lam K-W, Liu K, Yee R, Lee P: Detection of uric acid in aqueous humor by high pressure liquid chromatography. Curr Eye Res 2: 645-649, 1983.
8. Yonetani Y, Couzaki T, Ogawa Y: Epinepherine-induced hyperuricemia in experimental animals. Chem Pharm Bull 25: 441-447, 1979.
9. Bonney Ch, Lam K-W, Fong D: The integrity of the blood-aqueous barrier in hyperuricemia. Ann Ophth. In press.
10. Bonney Ch, Lam K-W, Fong D: Ocular hyperuricosis in the rabbit following hyperuricemia and topical epinepherine. J. Ocular Phar 2: 55-58, 1986.
11. Balentine JD: Principles of hyperoxic pathophysiology. In: Pathology of oxygen toxicity. Chapter 3: 31-81. Academic Press, New York, 1982.

Hyperbaric oxygen in the therapy of aphonia associated with chronic laryngitis

Philip B. James Ph.D., M.F.O.M.

Wolfson Institute of Occupational Health
The University of Dundee
Ninewells Medical School, Scotland, U.K.

SUMMARY

Although oxygen, given under hyperbaric conditions, has been shown to be effective in the control group of acute oedema, it has been difficult to accept that a rapid response may also be possible in a chronic state. A 40 year old patient with aphonia due to laryngitis has been treated for two separate episodes with oxygen delivered by mask at 2 ATA in a multiplace chamber. On both occasions his voice was restored by a single treatment of one hour. Additional therapy was required after a period of hours to restore the full benefit as the improvement began to recede. With each additional treatment the improvement remained for longer periods, mirroring similar findings in cerebral oedema. Laryngoscopy confirmed the presence of chronic oedema and the complete resolution, following a four day course of therapy, the first occasion. The second was tape-recorded using a standard technique before and after the first session of hyperbaric oxygen. The results indicate that the vasoconstriction obtained with hyperbaric oxygen can be of benefit in longstanding oedema, by breaking the vicious circle of hypoxia, oedema and microcirculatory insufficiency. The findings are applicable to other conditions associated with acute and chronic focal oedema, especially in the nervous system where oedema is so damaging.

CASE REPORT

The patient was a 40 year old practicing civil engineer and Deputy Principle of the University of Dundee. He had no history of serious illness and had never been hospitalized. His minor illnesses included herniation of an intervertebral disc and occasional sinus infections, usually following coryza. There had been a tendency for these episodes to be associated with loss of voice, but only for a day on any one occasion until 1985. On Friday the 4th of January 1985 he developed a cold and the following day his voice was reduced to a whisper. Four days later he consulted his general practitioner because of his laryngitis and continuing asphonia. No treatment was given on this or on a subsequent visit on the 15th of January. On the 25th of January he was prescribed an antibiotic by a dental practitioner and he was still unable to speak. He was seen by an otolaryngologist, who found odema in the vocal cords.

On the morning of the 6th of February, after being unable to speak for over four weeks, he was treated with hyperbaric oxygen by mask at 2 ATA in a multiplace chamber. There was almost full restoration of his voice after one hour. Because of a slight return of the discomfort with speaking, he received a second treatment on the same day and two subsequent session the following day, all at 2 ATA. This regime resulted in full recovery of his voice and the resolution of vocal cord oedema was confirmed by laryngoscopy.

He remained without symptoms until the 25th of September 1985, when he again lost voice after another coryzal infection. The first session of hyperbaric oxygen therapy, on the 30th of September, again restored his voice to a near normal level and tape recordings were made on a Sony Professional recorder before, during, and after the therapy. The waveform envelopes were displayed on a Tektronics 5103N storage oscilloscope. A dramatic difference in voice level was evident. Four sessions of hyperbaric oxygen therapy were undertaken, over the subsequent two days, to stabilize the benefit and the patient subsequently found that a further six sessions were helpful in controlling some recurring laryngeal discomfort.

DISCUSSION

The effect of therapy in this case was dramatic, but additional sessions were required to maintain the improvement. Because of the duration of the aphonia, the clinical condition can only be described as chronic, especially in the first episode, which lasted over four weeks. To find such a sudden reversal in long-standing tissue oedema is surprising and is likely to relate to the restoration of normal permeability in the micro-circulation and the improvement of lymphatic drainage. Virus may cause increased capillary permeability, but, in this patient, it is most unlikely that the causative virus would have persisted, especially in the first attack for weeks. It would seem probable that the increased permeability, caused by the original virus infection, led to focal oedema and the rise in tissue hydrostatic pressure prevented proper oxygenation by compressing the micro-circulation. As the respired gas passes over the vocal cords, the oxygen may be absorbed locally, as well as systematically. The effect should encourage us in the use of immediate oxygen therapy in a wide variety of conditions.

The reduction of oedema by hyperbaric oxygen is now well established scientifically, if not yet well known. Oxygen administered in this way provides the only method of reducing blood flow but, paradoxically, at the same time increasing oxygen in the control of acute oedema in other tissues, the most dramatic being in plastic surgery in the reduction of the oedema associated with pedicle flaps. In this situation the effect of a single treatment is usually not sufficient to ensure permanent resolution and benefit may not be sustained. It is, therefore, accepted that the therapy must involve serial exposures.

Although the value of hyperbaric oxygen therapy in nervous system disorders is yet to be widely accepted, oedema is a feature of both air embolism and decompression sickness. As research reveals the extent of the oedema, in dysbaric illness, the value of the correct partial pressure of oxygen in therapy is being recognized. Of course, the additional pressure required for hyperbaric oxygen therapy as the critical advantage of removing the causal gas phase in these conditions. In other nervous system disorders producing oedema the use of oxygen may not alter the underlying pathological disorder, but it is likely to minimize damage and buy crucial time for recovery, and argument first proposed by Haldane.

It is just as important to stress the need for serial exposures in the use of hyperbaric oxygen therapy in brain and spinal cord oedema, as it is in the healing of superficial wounds. The benefit of repeated therapy has been shown by serial measurements of intracranial pressure in patients with severe head injury, by Sukoff and Ragatz. Magnetic resonance imaging has now demonstrated that focal oedema is often present in apparently minor head injury, indicating the need for prophylactic treatment to prevent sequelae. It is clear that there is a scientific rationale for this approach in other conditions associated with focal oedema as, for example, in stroke and multiple sclerosis patients.

There are many accounts of sudden improvements, especially in bladder function, after a single treatment with hyperbaric oxygen in chronic multiple sclerosis patients, which mirror the restoration of voice in this case. Fortunately improvements in bladder function in multiple sclerosis patients have also been found under double-blind conditions 6,7,8,9. The effect emphasizes the need to treat episodes of focal oedema and dysfunction in the nervous system, from whatever cause with hyperbaric oxygen and as medical emergencies.

REFERENCES

1. Perrins DJD. Influence of hyperbaric oxygen on the survival of split skin grafts. Lancet 1967; i: 868-71.
2. Haldane JS. The therapeutic administration of oxygen. Brit Med J 1917; i: 183-185.
3. Sukoff M, Ragatz RE. Hyperbaric Oxygenation for the Treatment of Acute Cerebral Edema. Neurosurg 1982; 10: 29-38.
4. Gandy SE, Snow RB, Zimmerman RD, Deck MDF. Cranial nuclear magnetic resonance imaging in head trauma. Ann Neurol 1984; 16: 254-57.
5. Jenkins A, Teasdale G, Hadley MDM, Macpherson P, Rowan JO. Brain lesions detected by magnetic resonance imaging in mild and severe head injuries. Lancet 1986; ii: 445-446.
6. Fischer BH, Marks M, Reich T. Hyperbaric oxygen treatment of multiple sclerosis. New Eng J Med 1983; 308: 181-186.
7. Appell RA, Goodman JR, Deutsch JS. Van Meter K. Proceedings of the Urodynamics Society, Sixty Annual. Symp. New Orleans. May, 1984: 56.
8. Barnes MP, Bates D, Cartlidge NEF, French JM, Shaw DA. Hyperbaric oxygen and multiple sclerosis: short term results of a placebo-controlled, double-blind trial. Lancet 1985; i: 297-300.
9. Wiles CM, Clarke CRA, Irwin HP, Edgar EF, Swan AV. Hyperbaric oxygen in multiple sclerosis: a double blind trial. Brit Med J 1986; 292: 367-71.

The effect of hyperbaric oxygenation on the function of the adrenaline injured heart

Demurov E. A., Koloskov Yu. B. and Smurova T. G.

National Research Center of Surgery, Moscow, USSR

The lack of adequate criteria of HBO optimal regime providing the therapeutic effect and excluding toxic oxygen effect inhibits the rational use of HBO therapy for cardiovascular diseases. Taking into account the leading role of lipide peroxidation (LPO) in the oxygen pathogenesis we may suppose that the side effect of HBO on the heart might be due to the balance disturbance between the systems, activating and inhibiting LPO. It brings us to the idea that the use of antioxidants in combination with HBO will allow to expand the possibilities and increase the efficacy of HBO therapy for myocardial lesion.

The present paper describes the experiment on the model of adrenaline induced heart injury (AIHI) carried out to check the said supposition.

AIHI was produced in rabbits with the body mass 2.6 - 3.2 kg ay intravenous injection in 1% caffeine solution (20 mg/kg) and 0.1% adrenaline solution (0.3 ml) with 2 minute intervals. In the Control Group the animals received physiological solution.

The HBO sessions were initiated (2.5 ata, 1 hour) immediately after adrenaline infusion and were repeated every successive day. Left ventricle contractile function was accessed by the pressure in its cavity which was registered electromanomety by the polygraph "Minograph - 82" at rest and during 5 second occlusion of the ascending artery. Contraction and 5-second occlusion of the ascending artery. Contraction and myocardium relaxation velocity were also defined.

In the left ventricle tissue the activity of superoxide dismutase (SOD) was determined by the method based on the enzyme ability to inhibit adrenaline auto-oxidation. The anti-oxidant lipid activity (ALA) was also studied on the model of oxidation of methyl ether or oleine acid. The blood flow in the aorta was registered with a flowmeter.

In 2 hours after the cardiotoxic dose injection of adrenaline the rabbits showed the decrease in contractility and stroke volume. It was manifested in the decrease in left ventricle relaxation velocity at rest and stroke and minute cardiac output as compared to the Control Group by 20,30, and 21% correspondingly. At the same time there was a tendency to decrease in the developed pressure and left ventricle contraction velocity. During the experiment with aorta clamping the contractile cardiac function disturbance in animals with AIHI was even more pronounced. (fig.1)

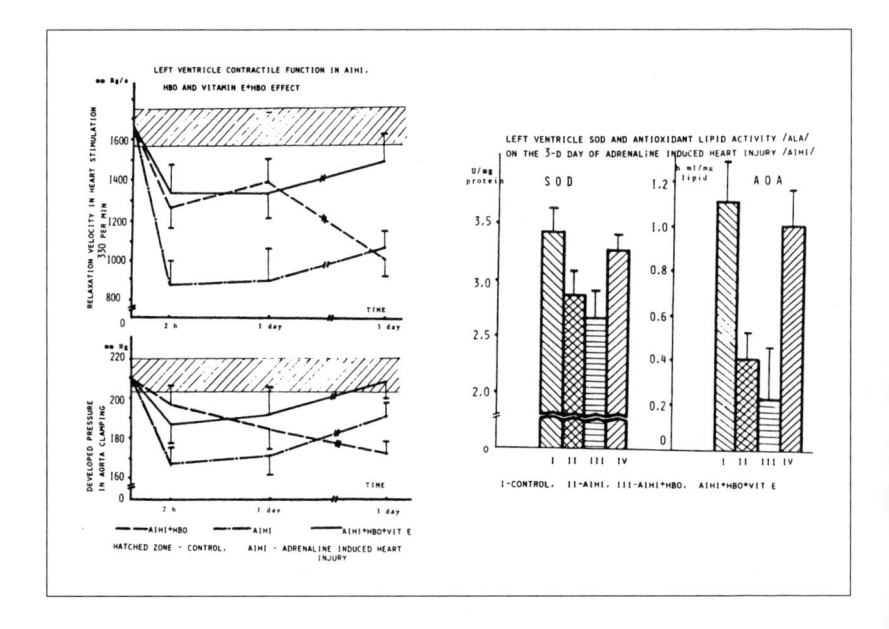

The sessions of HBO immediately following AIHI model prevented the fall in cardiac function in the majority of the studied parameters already on the 2nd hour. The HBO effect at rest was manifested in positive changes in cardiac output and relaxation velocity, and during aorta clamping the positive changes were observed in the developed pressure and relaxation velocity. The positive inotropic effect of HBO was still present 1 day after the AIHI modeling. During the next session of HBO on the third day of experiment the therapeutic effect was no longer observed and there were signs of oxygen toxic effect on the function and structure of cardiac muscle. The majority of cardiac contractility indices were on the lower level as compared to the Control Group of animals.

Two hours following the injection of necrosogenic dose of adrenaline in rabbits treated with HBO the signs of myocardial dystrophy and of myofibril and mitochondria destruction were less pronounced than in untreated animals. On the contrary, on the 3rd day of AIHI in rabbits treated with HBO glycogen in cardiomyocites and lysed myofibrils and vacuolated mitochondria were more frequently encountered.

Therapeutic effect of HBO on the function and structure of adrenergically damaged hear which was manifested in the course of the 1 day of pathologic process was realized on the background of higher (as compared to the Control Group) SOD activity and ALA myocardium. (fig.2)

Daily intramuscular infusion of natural antioxidant of vitamin E in a dose of 50 mg/kg during the whole period of experiment of the i/v injection of antioxidant SOD enzyme in a dose of 1 mg (2000 units) 3 times a day partially prevented the depression of cardiac contractility function in animals with AIHI on the third day of HBO therapy.

Vitamin E and SOD decreased the destructive changes in cardiomyocites in rabbits who had undergone the 3-day course of HBO after adrenaline injection. Protective effect of vitamin E against the oxygen toxic effect on the heart was accompanied by the increase in SOD and ALA in the left ventricle.

The cardiac activity in the rabbits with AIHI was changed in a quite different way when its antioxidant system was destabilized by the preliminary injection of SOD inhibitor DEDTC. Under the influence of DEDTC injected to the animals with AIHI undergoing the HBO therapy they have developed marked depression of cardiac contractility and pump function both at rest and in aorta clamping. In cardiomyocites of the left ventricle there was strongly pronounced fatty dystrophy and a great number of new formations such as: striped lipids, no glicogen, areas of hypercontraction and myofibrile lysis, mitochondria destruction, significant dilations of the sarcoplasmatic reticulum channels.

The data obtained shows that the combination of antioxidant drugs therapy and HBO treatment is the best method that provides positive results and protects against HBO toxic effect.

A transportable recompression chamber system

J. W. Pennefather

Royal Australian Navy School of Underwater Medicine
BALMORAL NSW 2091

ABSTRACT

A report of the development of a recompression chamber designed to be transportable by aircraft, truck and small boat.

The ergonomic considerations of the required patient care were used to decide the configuration. The resulting RCC is a truncated cone shape, length 2.3 meters; large diameter 1.12 meters; small diameter 0.44 meters. This provides space for the patient to sit or lie and for the attendant to examine and treat a recumbent patient.

The RCC can be inclined so that the patient is head down at 30°from horizontal. This is considered to reduce risk of re-embolisation in a patient with cerebral arterial gas embolism.

A carbon dioxide scrubber is fitted to reduce gas requirements. The scrubber can be air or electric drive. Electric drive is preferred for serious cases of decompression sickness as it allows control of oxygen pressure. Analyzers may be fitted to monitor oxygen and carbon dioxide concentration. A sealing ring around the door can be used to mate the RCC onto a compatible RCC. A small spherical RCC has been designed to gain the lock in advantage of two compartment RCC.

Other features include medical lock, communications system, gas supply and overboard exhaled gas dump system.

INTRODUCTION

Several Recompression Chambers are marked for the treatment and transportation of divers who have been injured far from a large recompression chamber. This new design originated as a design exercise after consideration of the problems in using these chambers for treating seriously ill divers. What was a paper exercise became a project following an approach to participate in the design of a chamber for the following uses:
    A. Therapeutic recompression of divers distant from a large recompression chamber.
    B. Transport of divers under pressure to a large chamber facility.

C. Surface decompression after dives.
D. Hyperbaric oxygen treatment when a large facility is not available.

A diver with serious decompression sickness or cerebral arterial gas embolism requires other treatment combined with recompression (1,2). He may also need restraining during oxygen induced convulsions. This care cannot be given in a one man recompression chamber.

Any change in recompression tables chosen is normally made as a result of neurological examination for evidence of incomplete recovery. Patients who don't recover may also need bladder catheterisation. Recent work on animals suggests that a patient with cerebral arterial gas embolism is best nursed in a head down posture (3). This position tends to prevent re-embolisation of the cerebral circulation. No transportable chambers are known to have space for the required neurological examination or to position a patient in a head down posture.

A list of ergonomic considerations was prepared outlining the features considered necessary:
A. Space is needed for the patient to sit or lie, a patient with air embolism is best nursed in a head down posture.
B. The attendant need to be able to reach all parts of the patient, he also needs a seat to rest on.
C. The panel operator and the placement of his controls needs to be planned, with consideration of space available in an aircraft.
D. The door and the chamber mating connections should be quick and easy to operate.

The reasons for the first two features are outlined above. The needs of the panel operator are more complex than in a fixed chamber because he may need to be strapped into an aircraft seat and still operate the chamber. The rapid closing of the door is a requirement for the conduct of surface decompression. The mating connection for joining the other chambers should also be easy to operate because it may be necessary to rapidly transfer attendants and patient to a larger chamber.

THE CHAMBER SYSTEM

The chamber is a truncated cone shape, it is 2.3 meters long with a maximum diameter of 1.12 meters. This shape allows space for the care needed. The patient can sit or lie on the litter. The attendant can reach the patient's toes, he has a folding seat adjacent to the patient's head. This folds back when extra space is needed.

The door remains inside the chamber. It is supported on a track and slide so that takes up the least possible space. The foot end of the chamber can be elevated for the treatment of patients with gas embolism.

The greatest difference between the chamber described and other chambers is facility to tilt to treat patients with air embolism. This is accomplished by lifting the foot end of the chamber. See Fig. 1.

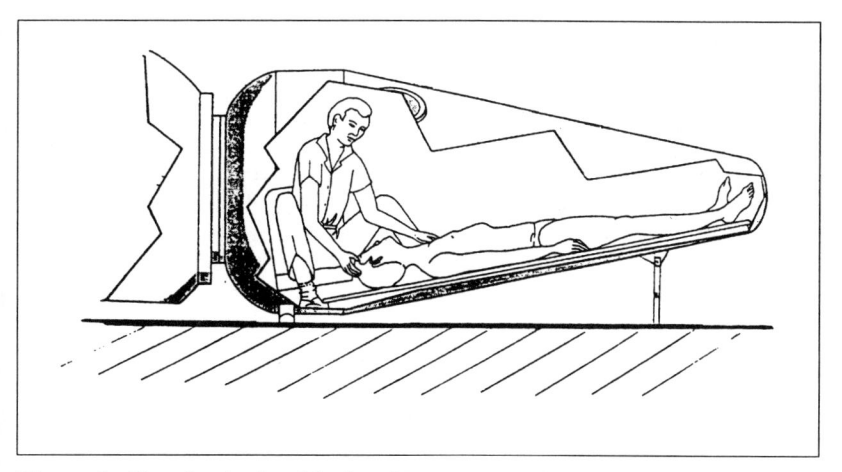

Figure 1. Chamber inclined for headdown posture in gas embolism treatment

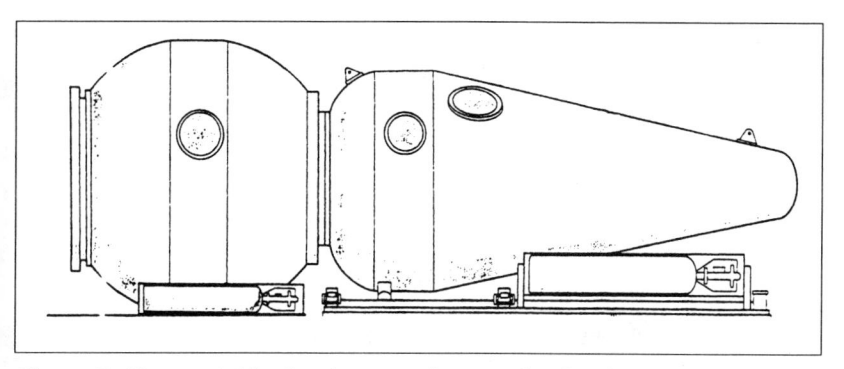

Figure 2. Transportable chamber mated to transfer chamber

    A carbon dioxide scrubber is fitted to reduce the air consumption. It is positioned outside the chamber so that the operator can service it. The external scrubber can be combined with heating or cooling for climate control. The standard scrubber is driven by a venturi system. If saturation treatments are contemplated the scrubber can be driven with an air/nitrogen mixture. An electrically drive scrubber could be fitted. This reduces air consumption. If it is used an oxygen analyzer would also be needed to ensure that the occupants did not suffer from hypoxia.

    Oxygen and carbon dioxide monitors can be fitted, these are highly desirable as a check that the occupants are given a safe breathing mixture. The oxygen analyses also provides a check that the oxygen dump system is working and that the masks are sealing properly.

The operator can be supplied with a remote console. With this he can operate the major controls and communicate with the occupants while he is seated near the chamber, this option should increase safety when the chamber is used in an aircraft. It should also reduce operator fatigue. He is also provided with an absolute pressure gauge connected to the chamber, this removes the need to correct for aircraft altitude during transport of a casualty.

The chamber can be locked on to other chambers that are fitted with a connecting flange. The N.A.T.O. connection is standard. Because the door of the transportable chamber does not protrude into the other chamber it can be locked onto chambers with a small outer lock. A smaller spherical chamber is being developed so that the chamber can be converted to a two compartment system when this is needed. See Fig. 2.

Exotic materials were considered for construction of the chamber. These are not acceptable under some pressure codes, some also have limited pressure ratings. For these reasons aluminum has been used.

PROGRESS REPORT

A mockup has been constructed to check the shape and size proposed. Fullerton Sherwood Ltd are constructing a prototype chamber based on the premises stated above, it is hoped to have it in Sydney for the Congress. Synergy Transfer of Sydney, Australia are handling sales enquiries.

REFERENCES:

1. Leitch DR, Green RD. Pulmonary baratrauma in divers and the treatment of cerebral gas embolism. Aviat. Space Environ. Med. 1986; 57:931-938.
2. Green RD, Leitch DR. Twenty years of treating decompression sickness. Aviat. Space Environ. Med in the press.
3. Gorman DF, Browning DM. Cerebral Vasoreactitivity and Arterial Gas Embolism Undersea Biomed. Res. 1986, 13;317-335.

Bronchial asthma treated by hyperbaric oxygen

A Report of 387 Cases

Wen-Ren Li, M.D.,

Fujian Provincial Hospital, Fuzhou, China;
Ly Zifan, Zhongshan Medical Centre, Guangzhou, China;
Yi Zhi, Guangzhou Hospital of Petrochemical Works, China.

Bronchial asthma is a common disease for which the choice of effective therapy is difficult because of its complex etiology. From 1976 to 1986 Hyperbaric Oxygenation was used as a trial to treat 387 patients suffering from the disease. The following is a summary of it.

CLINICAL MATERIALS

Of the 387 cases, 202 were male and 185 were female patients, mostly adults, and only 38 patients were under the age of 20. All have a clear diagnosis of bronchial asthma and have a history of 5-10 years of asphyxia attacks and have received various kinds of western and Chinese traditional therapy without any improvement and finally resorted to Hyperbaric Oxygenation therapy. The patients were treated with Hyperbaric Oxygenation of 2 ATA for 80 minutes with a break of 15 minutes between daily. One therapeutic course consisted of 24 treatments.

EVALUATION OF EFFICIENCY

Good results were obtained in 182 patients (47%), whose asphyxia attacks were decreased during the HBO treatment and ceased after the therapeutic course without taking broncholitic drugs and corticoid. The relief (free from attacks) period after a HBO course is over 6-12 months in 51 of the patients, and over one year in 69 of the 182 patients. (One course of HBO therapy is needed annually to strengthen the results).

Satisfactory results (decrease in frequency of asphyxia paroxysm and decrease in dosage of the drugs) were observed in 163 patients (42%). No effect was achieved in 42 patients (11%).

DISCUSSION

Mechanism of HBO Treatment

1) The etiology of bronchial asthma is complex. The studies in recent years show that allergy and functional disorder of vegetative nervous system are the two main factors in the development of the disease. Bronchial smooth muscle is controlled by both sympathetic and parasympathetic nerves (vagus). The excitement of vagus stimulates M-cholinergic receivers and activates guanosine cyclization enzyme, facilitating the formation of CGMP out of GTP in the cells, thus leading to a release of bioactivating agents, and so asphyxia paroxysms occur; moreover the bronchial relaxation and its stability is closely linked with physiological functions of CAMP, which stabilizes membrane potential of pulmonary smooth muscles and restrains the release of bioactivating agents, therefore making bronchi relax. CAMP is derived from ATP in the cells through catalysis of adenosine cyclization enzyme. A depressed function of adenosine cyclization enzyme and an insufficient amount of CAMP appeared in the body cells of patients with bronchial asthma. Therefore, most drugs used for relief of asphyxia attacks, e.g. adrenaline, aminophylline and corticoid have the property of enforcing the action of adenosine cyclization enzyme or raising the CAMP level by restraining its decomposition.

Under hyperbaric oxygenation there exists a higher level of metabolism within the body, a higher concentration of glucose in the blood as well as a favorable process of sugar, protein and adipose metabolism in the body cells, producing more ATP and CAMP; and the excited sympathetic nerves (due to HBO) will stimulate B-adrenergic receivers and so activate adenosine cyclization enzyme to change more ATP into CAMP, keeping the bronchi relaxed and stable.

2) During acute asphyxia paroxysms, the spasm of bronchial smooth muscle, swelling of bronchial mucous membrane and narrowing of the calibre of bronchi plus sputum trapped, will block airways and reduce the maximum ventilation volume and time vital capacity of the lungs. That is why in most cases of asphyxia attacks there exists anoxia and acidosis in different degrees. HBO treatment, however, can raise the tension, content and permeability of the blood oxygen considerably and so improve the hypoxic state of the local or systemic tissues and facilitate the repair of the affected bronchial tissues, alleviating congestion and swelling as well as spasms of the bronchial smooth muscles. There is one suggestion that oxygen in high density exerts a flush-sweep impact on the respiratory tract, reducing secretion of its glands and leaving the tract open, so that the vital capacity of the lungs will be promoted and symptoms like sense of a tight or heavy chest will be relieved. For reasons already mentions, some patients enjoy a longer period of freedom from attacks following HBO treatment.

3) Time Suitable for HBO Treatment, and its Contraindications. It was observed that some of the patients, if receiving HBO during their asphyxia attacks, felt tight in the chest and short of breath. This was because expiration becomes difficult under higher pressure. We recommend that HBO treatment be started during the attack-free period. In serious forms of the disease, if HBO (one or two treatments) is commenced every year before seasons of attack, a preventative effect may be achieved. HBO is not designed for those associated with severe pulmonary emphysema or huge sacs, in case of rupture of the alveoli or sacs, leading to pneumothorax. For those associated with pulmonary infection, antibiotics are advised in the prevention of spreading.

4) Because of its complex pathogenesis, bronchial asthma is difficult to cure despite efforts so far made with various western and Chinese traditional therapeutic agents. In many cases even temporary suspension of paroxysms is difficult. HBO therapy, however, not only ceases paroxysms within a short space of time but prevents recurrence for a longer period. This treatment should therefore be regarded as a new and promising method in coping with the disease. We recommend that all bronchial asthma be treated routinely with HBO if there are no contradictions.

Hyperbaric Medicine in China

Wen-Ren Li, M.D.,

People's Republic of China.

It is a great pleasure and honor for me to be invited by President Ian P. Unsworth to attend this IX International Congress on Hyperbaric Medicine. It will certainly provide me with an excellent opportunity to learn of recent advances and experiences from all these distinguished scholars and specialists in the field of Hyperbaric Medicine. I would now like to tell you something about the development of Hyperbaric Medicine in China.

In 1964 I successfully completed the construction and installation of an operating hyperbaric chamber, six meters in length and three meters in diameter, which was the first of its kind in China. After a series of animal experiments, I was able to arrest the heart successfully by inflow occlusion for about 30 minutes in the hyperbaric chamber at 3 ATA of oxygenation combined with mild hypothermia of 28-30°C. The long term survival rate of the experimental dogs was 86%. I then utilized the hyperbaric chamber at 3 ATA of oxygenation to treat tetanus, thromboangiitis obliterans, Raynaud's disease, sudden deafness, visual disturbances, hemiplegia due to cerebral artery thrombosis and various kinds of shock due to toxic lobar pneumonia, hemorrhage, myocardial infarction, etc., with gratifying results. In 1965 I could repair ventricular septal defect under HBO at 3 ATA combined with mild hypothermia of 28-30°C. In 14 of the 36 cases of congenital heart diseases operated on at 3 ATA of oxygenation, the period of complete circulatory arrest was more than 10 minutes. The boy with repair of ventricular septal defect stood very well and complete circulatory arrest of 20 minutes 16 seconds, with complete recovery. Follow-up studies showed that the boy has no neurological sequelae.

Open-heart surgery under extracorporeal circulation began rather late in the Fujian Province. From July 1965 until April 1966 I performed 15 open-heart operations under extracorporeal circulation at 3 ATA of oxygenation with only one death. I am sorry to say that this work was completely interrupted during the "Great Cultural Revolution." In 1973 we began to perform open-heart surgery again but progress was very slow. This was most unfortunate, as many important advances in hyperbaric medicine had been developed in the U.S., Japan, Europe and Australia during the interim seven years. After 1973, hyperbaric medicine in China gradually came to life, but the progress was slow before 1980. The Chinese Society of Hyperbaric Medicine was formally organized in August 1981, and I was elected President. It should be pointed out that all equipment used in hyperbaric medicine has been developed entirely from our own technical and material resources, as channels of international scientific exchange and purchase of equipment were not established then. In October 1983 I completed the construction and installation of a new large multiplace hyperbaric chamber, including an operating chamber, seven meters in length and four meters in diameter; a treatment chamber, six meters in length and three meters in diameter; and an air lock, three meters in diameter and 3.2 meters in height. On August 20, 1984, I presented a paper entitled "Open-heart surgery with extracorporeal circulation under hyperbaric oxygenation at 3 ATA - A report of 48 cases" at the VIII International Congress on Hyperbaric Medicine held at Long Beach, California, U.S.A. At present we treat about 30 patients with various diseases each day in the hyperbaric chamber, including multiple sclerosis, with very good results.

Aside from open-heart surgery being performed in the hyperbaric chamber, we have also performed a number of resections of esophageal carcinoma with transplantation of the transverse colon, subtotal and total gastrectomies, nephrectomies, resections of abdominal aortic aneurysm, and control of massive hemorrhage of the bile duct and gastrointestinal tract, using 3 ATA of hyperbaric oxygenation with satisfactory results.

In September 1965 I presented a paper entitled "The clinical application of hyperbaric oxygenation with a report of 64 cases" at the Conference of Cardiac Surgery in Shanghai. After the Conference physicians and surgeons from Beijing, Shanghai, Hangzhou, Guangzhou and Nanjing came to Fuzhou to investigate the feasibility of constructing a hyperbaric chamber in their hospitals. Since then hyperbaric chambers have been installed in various provincial hospitals in China. Up until now, there have been some 275 hyperbaric chambers spread all over China, even in Tibet we have four chambers (one large size chamber). Of the 275 chambers, 36 are multiplace, 49 are medium sized and 190 are monoplace chambers. The first National Conference on Hyperbaric Oxygenation was held in May 1973 in Hangzhou. The second National Conference was held in October 1979 in Guangzhou. The third was held in August 1981 in Qing-dao; the fourth in December 1984 in Fuzhou and the fifth, from September 26-29, was also held in Fuzhou. Fourteen outstanding professors, physicians, surgeons and specialists and their spouses, from as far afield as the U.S.A., Europe and Singapore, participated at the Fifth Conference.

Since 1979 the Chinese Society of Hyperbaric Medicine has staged a training course for physicians, surgeons and nurses undertaking hyperbaric oxygenation therapy. Until now we have trained six classes: in each class we have about 60-70 physicians and nurses and altogether have trained about 400 people.

We utilize the Hyperbaric Chamber to treat about 60 kinds of disease with very good results: with some of them we have achieved brilliant results. In China we have six factories able to design, construct and install hyperbaric chambers of varying sizes. We have composed a manual for physicians and nurses to follow during their HBO practice. The number of physicians, nurses and technicians practicing HBO exceeds 2000 and the number of patients receiving treatment exceeds 1,000,000. Our primary drawback is that we have very little research being done in the field of hyperbaric medicine, particularly in the fundamental theories of Hyperbaric Oxygenation. In order to promote Hyperbaric Medicine in China to the modern international level, and to meet with the great demand of our people, a team effort is required by Chinese physicians, surgeons, engineers, technicians and nurses. At the same time, we need more international exchange and assistance. As President of the Chinese Society of Hyperbaric Medicine, I would like to take this opportunity to welcome delegates from all countries to visit China and give us your kind support in promoting our level of Hyperbaric Medicine.

I wish to express my feelings of deep appreciation and gratitude to President Ian P. Unsworth and to the Chairman for giving me the opportunity to speak at this Conference.

I now propose that the venue for the X International Congress on Hyperbaric Medicine be held in the People's Republic of China in 1990, and I sincerely hope that the Governors of this Congress will approve my earnest request.

Hyperbaric oxygenation therapy for multiple sclerosis

A Report of 20 Cases

Wen-Ren Li M.D. and Zhou Xiu Zheng,

Fujian Provincial Research Institute for Cardiovascular Diseases,
Fuzhou, People's Republic of China

Multiple Sclerosis is a demyelinating disease of the central nervous system (CNS) which has a long chronic course, a high rate of disability and a tendency of progressively increasing morbidity. Up to now, people fail to get any definite effective treatment to this disease. Hyperbaric oxygenation (HBO) was used in 20 cases of this disease from 1985. We have achieved certain beneficial effects which will be reported as follows:
I. Standards for diagnosis: the diagnosis was according to the criteria of McDonald.
1. There are more than two foci in the CNS, such as the involvement of optic nerves, spinal cord, brain stem and cerebellum.
2. There are more than two times of remission, recurrences or stepwise aggravation during the whole course of the disease.
3. When the other lesions of the CNS have been excluded, the case meets the criteria of more than three items or two items of (1) and (3), or (2) and (3).
II. Clinical Materials:
Sex: Male patients - 12; Female patients - 8.
Age: Varies from 24-64 years.
Occurrence and Remote Cause: Seven cases of acute attack and 13 cases of chronic course; six cases in former and four cases in latter have the experiences of getting cold and trauma. No causes can be retraced in 10 cases. See Table 1 for symptoms and signs.
Foci of Involvement: Thirteen cases in the optic nerves, 13 cases in the brain stem, 11 cases in the cerebellum, five cases in the cerebrum and four cases in the spinal cord.
Adjuvant Examinations: Cerebro-spinal fluid examination revealed increasing IgG in six cases and oligoclonal band in four cases. CT scanning is 13 cases showed cerebral atrophy of varying degrees in six cases. High density calcified spots are found in the left temporal region and frontal lobes of the cerebrum in three cases. Only four cases are normal with CT scanning.

Evoked potential test revealed abnormal conductive route of optic nerves in five cases, of auditory nerves in four cases, normal in one case among the 10 cases receiving the examination. Abnormal somatosensory evoked potentials are not detected.

III. Treatment: The patients were treated in a big hyperbaric chamber. After the pressure of the chamber was increased to 2.5 ATA, the patient inhaled pure oxygen for 90 minutes with a break of 15 minutes, qd. The patients were treated 15-130 times. During the course of treatment, no hormone or other immunosuppressive drugs were given to the patients except for three cases of small doses of Dexamethasone used for a short period.

IV. Evaluation of the Effects: if the symptoms and signs disappear, the patient is classified as completely relieved. If the symptoms get better and the signs disappear partially, then the patient is classified as markedly improved. If the patient feels better but without any marked reduction of signs, then he is classified as improved. The patient without any improvement in symptoms and signs is classified as no effect. If both symptoms and signs are aggravated then the patient is classified as deteriorated. The result of these 20 cases treated with HBO: one case completely relieved; eight cases markedly improved; seven cases improved; four cases no effect. There was no case deteriorated. Among the eight cases of marked improvement, the auditory evoked potential improved in two cases, and the optic evoked potential improved in two cases. These correspond very well with the marked improvement in the clinical symptoms.

DISCUSSION

Multiple sclerosis is now generally considered to be an immunological disease of the CNS. Pathologically it is characterized by the demyelination and gliosis in the white matter. It usually involves the optic nerves, spinal cord, brain stem, cerebellum and cerebrum. Because of the axonal preservation in the early stage of the disease, the demyelination can repair itself which accounts for the self-relief of the symptoms and signs. But the disease recurs easily and it seems a long, chronic course, resulting in visual impairment, paralysis, ataxia, dysarthria and other severe sequelae which lead to disability or death due to severe complications. Through immunology, electrophysiology and radiology, early diagnosis can be made, depending on the increasing IgG index and oligoclonal band from cerebrospinal fluid examination, abnormal evoked potential (visual, auditory and somatosensory) and CT scanning, even if the clinical appearance is atypical. Through the test of nuclear magnetic resonance, the diagnosis of MS will be made more accurate. With regard to treating disease, it is still a problem. Many investigators have been devoted to the research of immunosuppressive treatment for over 20 years. Though effective control on acute attacks has been shown by a short course of a large dose of hormonal treatment, there is no evidence to suggest that it can prevent recurrence of the disease, nor reduction in its severity. Other treatment such as transfer factor cyclophamicle and lymphocytapheresis have not given convincing results.

Animal experiments suggest that HBO therapy may have the effect of immunosuppression by decreasing the size of the spleen and the amount of lymphocyte in the circulation, by lengthening the life of transplanted skin and suppressing the experimental allergic cerebrospinitis. HBO therapy can relieve the anoxic state of nerve tissue, retard the breakdown of myelin due to inflammation, and hasten the repair of oligodendrocyte. Although this has not been clinically proven, there is evidence to suggest that HBO therapy has enough theoretical basis for the treatment of multiple sclerosis.

In this group of 20 cases of HBO therapy, four cases failed to improve. The total effective rate was 80%. Case four, whose course was eight months, developed diplopia, nystagmus, ataxia, hemiparesis in the right limb and dysarthria during an acute attack. The symptoms and signs could not be controlled during the first 12 HBO therapy treatments. Following intravenous Dexamethoni 4 mg being added every day for 13 days, and a further 80 HBO treatments, the patient was completely relieved. It is worth mentioning that patients with MS often have severe symptoms and signs, long course, who received hormonal treatment for long periods, usually have a high morbidity rate and often die of side effects of hormonal therapy such as infection. HBO therapy can increase the survival rate by avoiding these effects. From 1977-1982, we treated seven cases of MS, courses varying from five to nine years. They received high doses of hormone therapy during their attacks. Amongst the seven patient, five died. Case 17 was a man aged 40 with severe symptoms and signs of MS for three years. When admitted to our hospital he had more severe symptoms and signs than the other six, with loss of consciousness, spastic paralysis in four extremities, zero degree myodynamia, aphagia, and incontinence of both urine and stool. Following a small dose of hormone during the acute stage, he was treated with HBO therapy for 130 sessions. He regained consciousness, with improvement of myodynamia and reduction of muscle spasm. He began to walk with help, and fed himself. Reexamination of the patient revealed marked improvement in the optic and auditory conduction routes. Although we are unsure, we feel that HBO therapy with a small dose of hormone was beneficial in treating this acute case.

The results showed the HBO therapy could produce better effects on MS when the disease course is short. In the acute stage of the disease, when there is brain inflammation and edema, a small dose of hormone should be added to the HBO therapy. Patients with longer course and more recurrences usually have irreversible scoliosis and the effect of HBO therapy is unsatisfactory. In some patients, although the course of the disease is longer, certain improvement can be obtained because of the presence of partial remaining axon in the severe demyelinating nerve tissue. There is something worth mentioning in that case nos. 1 and 17 usually felt better following each course of HBO therapy. This shows that there is a lasting beneficial effect from HBO therapy on repairing the myelogene, thereby decreasing the chance of recurrence. The question of whether HBO therapy can change the course of the disease remains open.

Myasthenia gravis treated by hyperbaric oxygenation

A Report of 40 Cases

Wen-Ren Li, M.D., Li Jien Chen and Zhe Feng Jing

P.R., China.

Myasthenia Gravis is a disease characterized by weakness of the ocular and other cranial nerve innervated muscles, with no signs of neural lesion, and partial reversibility by the administration of either cholinergic drugs or inhibitors of the enzyme cholinesterase. There is evidence to suggest that this is an autoimmune disorder. The basic defect which is focused on the receptor for acetylcholine by a specific antibody has been indicated recently. Since steroids and immunosuppressive drugs revealed a good response in some cases of myasthenia gravis, we were encouraged to commence a trial using Hyperbaric Oxygenation in the treatment of this disease.

CLINICAL MATERIALS

Forty patients with myasthenia gravis were treated with Hyperbaric Oxygenation (HBO) from October 1982 to December 1985. There were 18 males and 22 female patients with an average history of 3.2 years duration. There were 26 cases involving the ocular muscles, 10 were generalized, and four involved bulbar myasthenia gravis. They had all received neostigmine or pyridostigmine except for one case of thymectomy. Twenty eight cases had received dexamethasone. The patients were admitted to the hospital because of exacerbation of the illness or failure to respond to drug therapy. Diagnosis was further confirmed by serial examinations. Patients were randomly divided into three groups:

Group A: Eighteen patients treated with HBO at 2.5 ATA for one hour q.d. ALONE, and 30 days for one therapeutic course.

Group B: Twenty two cases treated with HBO at 2.5 ATA for one hour q.d., combined with Dexamethasone 10-20mg q.d. for 15-20 days, then gradually tapered to maintenance dose.

Group C: Twenty cases roughly matched with Groups A and B for age and sex treated with Dexamethasone alone to serve as a control.

EVALUATION OF THE THERAPEUTIC RESPONSE

EXCELLENT
Toxicity of the involved muscles recovered completely to normal and were able to do daily work, without recurrence for at least one year following HBO therapy.

GOOD
Symptoms and signs disappeared or were greatly relieved.

NO EFFECT
Symptoms and signs persisted without improvement.

RESULTS
The short term therapeutic response implied that the response was evaluated after completion of the therapeutic course, while the long term response was the evaluation of the response at a period of six months to three years following cessation of the therapeutic course.

SHORT TERM EVALUATION
In Group A (HBO therapy alone), 15 of the 18 cases (83%) had excellent response, while the remaining three (16.6%) had a good response. In Group B (HBO with Dexamethasone), there were 20/22 cases (91%) with an excellent response, and the remaining two with a good response. In Group C (Dexamethasone alone), 11 of the 20 cases (55%) had an excellent response, six (30%) responded well and three (15%) were not affected.

LONG TERM EVALUATION
In Group A (HBO therapy alone) there were 14/18 cases (78%) with excellent response, two (11%) with good response and two (11%) with no effect. In Group B (HBO with Dexamethasone) 17/22 cases (77%) were excellent, two (9%) were good, and three (14%) were not affected. In Group C (Dexamethasone alone) four of the 20 cases (20%) had an excellent response, five (25%) had a good response and 10 (50%) were not affected. The symptoms and signs of one case (5%) worsened.

DISCUSSION

Myasthenia Gravis is an autoimmune disease. The elevation of serum and cerebrospinal fluid IgG in these patients has been noted. It was recently reported that a specific antibody against the receptor of acetylcholine had been found in 85% of patients with MG and that the major component of this antibody is IgG. HBO therapy revealed an effect on the concentration of serum immunoglobulins, particularly in IgG. Reduction of serum IgG by HBO was found in animal experimentation and clinical observation. These findings suggest that HBO may affect immunosuppression of the organism. The preliminary results of our trial indicate that HBO therapy is of benefit to MG sufferers, its effectiveness approaching 100% in the short term and 87.5% in the long term. The response of 18 patients using HBO therapy alone was much better than those using Dexamethasone only. Patients usually recovered completely and led active daily lives following completion of HBO therapy alone without the need to take drugs. It is worthwhile mentioning that the response of HBO with Dexamethasone in Group B was superior to that of Group A (HBO alone). HBO therapy reduced the side-effects of Dexamethasone and the transient exacerbation of the illness at the beginning of Dexamethasone therapy alone. The combination of HBO with Dexamethasone might have had a synergic effect on the response.

The effects of high pressure of N2 and He on neurotransmitter (dopamine) release from rat striatum

R. B. Philp and M. L. Paul,

Department of Pharmacology and Toxicology,
University of Western Ontario, London Ontario,
CANADA N6A 5C1.

INTRODUCTION

The narcotic properties of inert gases such as nitrogen (N2) have long been known and impose depth limitations upon diving with compressed air. A rule-of-thumb, known somewhat facetiously as "Martini's Law" holds that each 15m of seawater produces narcosis equivalent to the intoxicating effect of one martini (1). This phenomenon has necessitated the substitution of helium (He) for N2 as the inert component of the breathing mixture for dives in excess of 60-70m. As depth limits were gradually pushed back, a new neurological problem emerged. Known as the High Pressure Neurological Syndrome (HPNS), it consists of an array of signs that include tremor (at 8-12Hz), muscle fasciculations, myoclonic jerks, decrement in psychomotor performance, dizziness, nausea, vomiting, impaired consciousness and dyspnea (1). The apparently-opposing effects of Inert Gas (N2), Narcosis and HPNS led to the employment of an He/N2/02/ breathing mixture, called Trimix, which indeed controls the disorder and which has commercial operations. Nevertheless, HPNS remains the limiting factor for deep-sea diving.

The effects of pressure and N2 obviously must both operate through some, possibly the same, site or sites in the CNS, lending appeal to the search for a common basis of explanation. At present, the most attractive hypothesis is the "critical volume hypothesis," first proposed by Miller as a mechanism for explaining the action of anesthetic agents (2). According to this theory, anesthetics, including N2 expand the plasma membranes of neurons, rendering them insensitive to the events necessary for the transmission of impulse waves. Conversely, pressure would compress the membrane to generate, if not opposite, at least different physiological effects. Credence is given to this proposition by the fact that pressure has been shown to reverse the effects of anesthetics under several experimental conditions. These studies have been reviewed by Halsey (3).

Neural defects that have been shown to occur in experimental HPNS include slowing of axonal conduction and prolongation of the action potential, depression of synaptic transmission and inconsistent effects on brain levels of various neurotransmitters (3). In an effort to investigate more closely the effects of pressure and of N2 on neurotransmitter release and metabolism in the system less vulnerable to the complexities of whole-brain analysis, we have been studying the release of dopamine and its metabolites from isolated tissue of rat brain striatum, and some preliminary findings are reported herein.

METHODS

Bilateral striata were rapidly excised from the brains of adult male Sprague-Dawley rats (350g) following decapitation. The tissue was mechanically sliced using a tissue slicer designed by Bennett and colleagues (4) to yield 400 x 400um sections which were transferred to the stainless steel perfusion cuvette. The preparation was superfused at a rate of 1.0ml/min. with zero-Ca++ Krebs-buffer for 30 min. prior to sample collection. "Baseline" release of neurotransmitters was initiated by substituting normal Krebs medium containing (mM) 120NaCl, 4.75KCl, 1.2KH2PO4, 1.2MgSO4, 25NaHCO3, 2.6CaCl2 and 10 Glucose. Throughout the experiment, all superfusion media were equilibrated with 95% O2/5%CO2 and kept at 37°C (pH 7.4). Two ml. samples were collected in tubes chilled to 4°C and containing 60ul of 2NHCl with the internal standard dihydroxybenzylamine (DHBA). The final pH of the sample was 2.5-3.5. "Evoked" release was measured by changing to Krebs with elevated K+ (35 or 60mM: the mM of NaCl was reduced accordingly).

Experiments were conducted in 1 ATA air, 48 ATA He or N2 and 100 ATA He. The design of the hyperbaric chamber requires a minimum driving pressure to facilitate collection of the perfusate so that in the He and N2 experiments, "baseline" samples were initially collected at 2 ATA as well as during and after compression at 10 ATM/min. "Evoked" release was measured after reaching 48 ATA. In all experiments, compression with inert gas was instituted over 1 ATA of air in the chamber.

Following decompression (and at the end of the 1 ATA experiment) the tissue was recovered and homogenized by sonication in an acetate-perchloric acid medium of the following composition: 0.5M acetic acid, 0.5M Na acetate, 04M HClO4, 25ng/ml DHBA, pH 4.8.

The sample was clarified by centrifugation at 12 000 x G for 30 min. at 4°C and the supernatant was kept for HPLC analysis of "residual" transmitter content. The pellet was stored at -80°C for subsequent protein analysis using the Lowry method (5). Compounds of interest were quantified using reverse-phase HPLC with electrochemical detection. These included the "parent" amines, noradrenaline, adrenaline, dopamine (DA), 5-hydroxytryptamine, and metabolites 3, 4-dihydroxyphenylacetic acid (DOPAC), 3-

methoxy-4-hydroxyphenylacetic acid (HVA), 3-methoxytyramine (3 MT), 5-hydroxy-3-indole acetic acid (5HIAA) and 5-hydroxytryptophol (5HTOL).

RESULTS

Of the compounds noted above, only DA and DOPAC were consistently detected in the superfusate collected from striatal tissue. Throughout the initial perfusion period with normal Krebs medium there was a measurable efflux of DOPAC while DA was only seen in some samples and at lower levels. Switching to 35 or 60mM K± Krebs promoted a rapid burst of DA release which usually reached maximum within the first 2 min. and then immediately began to decline. DOPAC levels also increased following K± induced depolarization and the maximum was seen 2-3 min. following the DA peak. The limit of detection for DA and DOPAC was approximately 05.ng/mg of protein.

K+ was superfused continuously for 15 min. as a 60 or 35mM solution,a and also for 6 min. continuously, or as two, 6 min. intermittent pulses of 35mM. The last has been selected as evoking satisfactory depolarization with minimal risk of tissue damage. To date, 2-4 experiments have been conducted at each pressure, gas and K+ combination.

In Table 1 the total output of DA and DOPAC are shown, together with their residual tissue levels, for the various experimental conditions. In all experiments, the release of DA and DOPAC was directly proportional to both the duration and strength of the stimulus (K+). Exposure to 48 ATA of N2 consistently depressed total output of DA and DOPAC under all experimental conditions. No consistent pattern regarding residual levels of either DA or its metabolite were noted.

Results with He were more variable. Reduced release of DA was observed at 48 ATA when the K+ stimulus was 60mM for 15 min. or in one or two pulses of 35mM, but was greater than control (1 ATA air) at 35mMK+ for 15 min. At 100 ATA of He, DA output was consistently higher than controls in these experiments performed to date. Residual levels of DOPAC were consistently much lower than those at 1 ATA of air.

DISCUSSION

There is now convincing evidence that over 90% of DA released from stratium is synthesized novo in response to wave impulse generation (6). Since DOPAC, whether released or residual, reflects biotransformation of DA by monoamine oxidase (7), the sum of released DA plus released and residual DOPAC is a reasonable reflection of total DA synthesis. Granule stores of DA appear not to contribute much to released neurotransmitter. There is little doubt, therefore, that the synthesis of DA was inhibited by 48 ATA of N2. To take but one example (60mMK+) this sum for 1 ATA air is 186ng/mg protein, vs. 122 for N2. This evidence of depressed synthesis need not reflect suppression of enzyme activity but could result from impaired movement of substrate (dihydroxphenylalanine) within the neuron since this is synthesized both in the cell body and the nerve terminal (7). Depression of neurotransmitter availability is compatible with the narcotic action of N2. So far, the results with He are inconclusive. There is a suggestion that it may actually increase neurotransmitter release, which would be in keeping with the excitatory effects of pressure in HPNS, but this requires confirmation.

Even if inert gas narcosis and HPNS operate through a common target such as the cell membrane, as the critical volume hypothesis implies, the interpretation of their behavioral and physical effects will remain difficult. Recently we reported on a study of the effects of compressed air on drug-induced stereotyped behavior and locomotion in mice (8). Both activities involve dopamine receptor systems but whereas increased locomotor activity induced by d-amphetamine and morphine was significantly potentiated by compressed air, stereotyped behavior was generally depressed, which cannot adequately be explained y a general depression of dopamine release. One possibility is that perturbations of membranes could induce changes in the configuration of neurotransmitter receptors. Using platelet aggregation as a model we have shown that both N2 and pressure alter the response of platelets to receptor-mediated stimuli of aggregation (9). The present study however, strongly implicates depressed neurotransmitter release as playing a role in inert gas narcosis.

Table 1. Total release of dopamine and dopac and residual striatal levels (ng/mg protein) during and after K± evoked depolarization under various conditions of gas, pressure and stimulus strength residual levels shown in brackets.

GAS	ATA	mMK+ and (Time, min.)			
		60(15)	35(15)	35(6+6)	35(6)
A. DOPAMINE					
Air	1	70(55)	26(51)	20(43)	14(NA)
N2	48	59(50)	20(57)	11(42)	7(NA)
He	48	66(41)	28(69)	15(31)	11(NA)
	100	—	—	—	25(NA)
B. DOPAC					
Air	1	81(35)	52(25)	47(11)	30(NA)
N2	48	40(23)	27(14)	32(12)	23(NA)
He	48	52(15)	45(14)	35(8)	25(NA)

ACKNOWLEDGEMENT

Supported by a research contract from the Canadian Defense and Civil Institute of Environmental Medicine, Downsview, Ontario.

REFERENCES

1. Edmonds, C., Lowry, C. and Pennefather, J. Diving and Subaquatic Medicine. Diving Medical Centre Publ., Sydney, 1983.
2. Miller, K.W. Inert gas narcosis, the high pressure neurological syndrome, and the critical volume hypothesis. Science 185:867, 1974.
3. Halsey, M.J. Effects of high pressure on the central nervous system Physiol. Rev. 62:1341, 1982.
4. Bennett, G.W., Sharp, T.A., Marsden, C.A. and Parker, T.L. A manually-operated brain tissue slicer suitable for neurotransmitter release studies. J. Neurosci. Meth. 7:107, 1983.
5. Cooper, J.R., Bloom, F.E., and Roth, R.H. The biochemical basis of neuropharmacology. Chap. 7, Oxford University Press (Lond.), 1982.
6. Lowry, O.H., Rosenbrough, N.J., Lewis-Fair, A. and Randall, R.J. Protein measurement with the Folin phenol reagent. J. Biol. Chem. 193:265, 1951.
7. Herdon, H., Strupish J. and Nahorski, S.R. Differences between the release of radiolabelled and endogenous dopamine from superfused rat brain slices: Effects of depolarizing stimuli, amphetamine and synthesis inhibition. Brain Res. 348:309, 1985.
8. McIlwain, H. and Bachelard, H.S. Biochemistry and the Central Nervous System. Chap. 15: Amines associated with neurotransmission. Churchill Livingstone, N.Y., 1985.
9. Philp, R.B., Fields, G.N.D. and Johnston, J.J. Effects of nitrogen and helium at pressure on drug-induced stereotypy and locomotion in mice. Aviation, Space, Environ. Med. 57:769, 1986.
10. Philp, R.B. Fields, N. and McIver, D.J.L. Interaction of high pressure and anaesthetics on blood platelet function. Undersea Biomed. Res. 12 (Suppl): 36(Abst.), 1985.

Hyperbaric oxygen and vasodilating therapy for idiopathic sudden hearing loss

Goto F., Sasaki M., Kato K.a and Fujita T.

Gunma University Hospital
Maebashi, Gunma, Japan

The cause of idiopathic sudden hearing loss is thought to be vascular or viral in origin, resulting in reduced blood and oxygen supplies to cochlea. However, there does not seem to be any agreement among otolaryngologists regarding treatment for sudden hearing loss. Many researchers have reported varying degrees of success of treatment through the use of a number of compounds such as vasodilators, anticoagulants, vitamins, steroid hormones and tranquilizers.

Appaix (1), Lamm (2) and Yanagita (3) have reported better results in patients treated with hyperbaric oxygen (HBO) therapy, than in patients treated with vasodilators or antiinflammatory drugs. Conversely, constriction of cerebral blood vessels upon induction of oxygen was reported. Murata et al (4) reported that depressed cochlear microphonics due to HBO induction was allayed with the resection of the superior cervical ganglion in animals.

This report is a presentation of the results from a series of studies on HBO combined with stellate ganglion block (SGB) in order to inhibit constriction of blood vessels due to induction of HBO (5).

Moreover, prostaglandin E_1 (PGE_1) drip infusion has been combined with SGB and HBO therapy in order to make sure of the vasodilating action. This treatment is considered to be effective for patients who were treated two weeks after the onset of the symptoms.

MATERIALS AND METHODS

The typical patient is one who suddenly becomes hard of hearing or deaf in one ear for no apparent reason. Conditions that are known to produce abrupt and unilateral sesorineural hearing losses, such as mumps, measles, acoustic tumors, ear surgery, head injury, ototoxic drugs and explosion were excluded from this case report.

Group 1 patients were treated with dexamethasone, vitamin B, kallidin and nucleoside. These patients did not receive SGB and HBO therapy because of personal reasons.

SGB and HBO therapy (Group II) and SGB and HBO combined with PGE_1 infusion (Group III) were employed for 65 and 63 patients, respectively. All patients were informed of the nature of treatment in detail and written consent was obtained prior to the initiation of therapy.

The SGB procedure incorporated was Moor's anterior approach: (6) and the technique consists of an injection of 6 to 8 ml 0.35% bupivacaine. The patients were observed until the onset of Horner syndrome. Group III patients received PGE_1 (60ug in 200ml lactated Ringer solution) drip infusion for 30 min following SGB.

Group II and Group III patients were exposed to oxygen pressure of 2.0 ATA for 60 min. Each patient was routinely treated 20 times during a period of 4 weeks. Once a week, patients were re-evaluated audiologically. When patients recovered completely within 20 treatments, the therapy was stopped. Patients who indicated that significant recovery continued after 20 treatments were

Hearing level recovery rates were compared by examination of the audiogram from the first day to the last, during our study.

Hearing was considered to have improved significantly when recovery of pure tone average (250-400 Hz) of over 10dB was attained. Patients whose audiogram stabilized within 20dB of hearing loss were considered to have recovered normal hearing ability.

Student's test was used for statistical analysis with a P value of less than .05 considered to represent a statistically significant change. Data are expressed as mean ± SEM.

RESULTS

The average age of patients was 40 years. 52% were men and 48% women. There were no significant differences between three groups in average age and sex. Every patients treated within one week following the onset of symptoms had good results. However, in group I, patients treated later than one week following the onset of symptom were treated two weeks or more following the onset of symptom were treated two weeks or more following the onset. In Group II and III, the rate of improvement in the patients treated within 2 weeks following the onset was almost similar, but there was a significant difference (P<0.05) between group II and group III in the 2nd-4th week bracket (table 1). In group III, 73% (8/11) of the patients improved compared to 42% (5/12) in group II.

Table 2 shows the age at the onset of symptoms. The rate of improvement in the over 40 years bracket was significantly low (p<0.05). In the under 40 age bracket 95% (19/20) patients exhibited pure tone improvement of over 10dB in group III and a 34 year old male patient recovered normal hearing level after 4 weeks following the onset of symptoms. One younger patient who did not have any improvement was total hearing loss type.

DISCUSSION

Shaia and Sheehy (7) reviewed 1200 cases and reported the effect of medical treatment with vasodilators for 380 patients. Of the treated group,

40% exhibited significant hearing improvement. There was a direct relationship between the time of onset of treatment and the number of patients who showed improvement.

Haug et al. (8) reported the effect of SGB and Yanagita et al. reported good results following treatment with HBO. However, the incidence of significant pure tone improvement in patients treated two weeks after the onset was no so high. Our study shows that there is a 91% chance that patients treated within 2 weeks after the onset will recover over 10dB, and a 50% (44/88) chance that almost normal hearing level will be regained in group II and III. Moreover, 48% patients treated later than 2 weeks to 2 months following the onset achieved over 10dB pure tone improvement.

Age is also an important factor. Patients under 40 years old almost always improve even when the initiation of treatment was delayed in the study, except one case who had complete deafness. Two cases treated after 4 weeks recovered in the under 40 bracket.

During the last five years most patients who suffered from sensorineural hearing loss were treated with PGE_1 infusion and/or HBO plus SGB. We believe that SBG and HBO therapy is effective in the treatment of sudden idiopathic hearing loss (5). However, there is no agreement among otolaryngologists and anesthesiologists regarding another vasodilating therapy such as oral drug therapy and/or PGE_1 infusion is necessary or not during SGB and HBO therapy.

From the data cited here and former report (5) it would seem appropriate to further expand the application of SGB and HBO accompanied by drug therapy and/or PGE_1 infusion to patients who receive their treatment more than two weeks following the onset of hearing loss.

Table 1. Pure Tone Average Improvement (250-4000Hz) in Patients Treated with Medical Treatment (Group 1), SGB and HBO (Group II) and SGB and HBO combined with PGE1 infusion (Group III).

Interval before Treatment <day>	Group	No	Complete Recovery	Pure Tone Improvement over 30dB	29-10dB	9-0dB	Improved Cases <%>
1~7	I	13	1	4	4	4	69
	II	24	1	8	12	3	88
	III	20	4	8	7	1	95
8~14	I	9	0	0	3	6	33
	II	17	0	7	8	2	88
	III	27	2	14	9	2	93
15~21	II	11	2	1	2	6	46
	III	8	0	2	4	2	75
22~28	II	1	0	0	0	1	0
	III	3	0	0	2	1	67
29~60	II	12	1	0	4	7	42
	III	5	1	0	0	4	20

Table 2. Age at Onset of Symptoms in Group III

Age	No	Complete Recover	Pure Tone Improvement over 30dB	29-10dB	9-0dB	Improved Cases <%>
6~19	12	0	8	3	1	92
20~39	18	4	8	6	0	100
40~59	22	1	7	9	5	77
60~79	10	2	1	4	3	70

REFERENCES

1. Appiax A, Peach A, Demard F: L'utilisation de l'oxygene hyperbare en oto-rhino-laryngologie. Ann Otolaryngol Chir Cervico-Fac (Paris) 87:7355, 1970.
2. Lamm H, Klimpel L: Hyperbare Sauerstoff therapie bei Innenohr-und Vestibularisstorungen. HNO 19:363, 1971.
3. Yanagita N, Miyake II: Sudden deafness and hyperbaric oxygen therapy. Clinical report of 25 patients. Fourth International Hyperbaric Congress Proceedings p389, 1974.
4. Murata K, Takeda T, Iwai H: Cochlear microphonics in oxygen at high pressure. Arch Otorhinolaryngol 208:77, 1974.
5. Goto F, Fujita T, Kitani Y, et al: Hyperbaric oxygen and stellate ganglion blocks for idiopathic sudden hearing loss. Acta Otolarygol 88:335, 1979.
6. Moor DC: Anterior approach for block of the stellate ganglion. Regional block anesthesia. 4th ed. Charles C Thomas Pub. Springfield p123, 1965.
7. Shaia FT, Sheehy JL: Sudden sensorineural hearing impairment: A report of 1220 cases. Laryngoscope 85:389, 1975.
8. Hang D, Draper Wl, Hang SA: Stellate ganglion blocks for idiopathic sensorineural hearing loss. Arch Otolaryngol 102:5, 1976.

Hyperbaric oxygen therapy for central nervous disorders

PET (positron emission tomography) study

Yasuharu Kitani, Katoko Miura,
Yoshitaka Uchihashi and Tatsushi Fujita;

Department of Anesthesiology, School of Medicine,
Gunma University, Maebashi, Gunma 371, Japan.

We begin the clinical application of measuring local cerebral functions with the reconstruction of PET images through the inhalation of oxygen (15 0) labed isotopes, carbon dioxide (C15 02), and oxygen (15 O2) gases in April 1984. Using the Japan Steelworks manufactured AVF (flat convergence) cyclotron located at Gunma University, the preparation of these radiopharmaceuticals was relatively easy to produce (1, 2).

As for hyperbaric oxygen therapy (HBO therapy), its expectations for treating central nervous disorders have grown in recent years. At the same time, testing methods that disclose the morbid state are awaiting to examine the therapeutic efficacy of HBO therapy. In this study, HBO therapy was performed on two typical cases of carbon monoxide poisoning (CO poisoning) referred for HBO therapy and two cases with cerebrovascular impairment following cardiac arrest revival, whereupon the efficancy of HBO therapy was examined by PET.

SUBJECTS AND METHOD

Subjects

The subjects involved two cases with CO poisoning referred to the Gunma University Hospital for HBO therapy and two cases with cerbrovascular impairment following cardiac arrest revival.

Method

In addition to morphological imaged by X-Ray CT, the electroencephalograph (EEG) was also recorded by the EEG topographic map as an electrophysiological method of examination. The regional cerebral blood flow (rCBF) was measured by C15 O2 inhalation and the regional cerebral metabolic rate (rCMRO2) by 15 O2 inhalation employing the Hitachi positron CT (PCT-H1) for the head region. A comparative study was then undertaken on the produced images. For each subject scanning before and after treatment of HBO was conducted during continuous inhalation. Two arterial samples were taken during scanning and information derived quantitative rCMRO2 and rCBF.

RESULTS

Case I: Aged 32 years; male. The subject attempted suicide by inhaling gas exhaust from a car. He was found in a coma and taken to a hospital where a crisis was indicated. Pharmacotherapy using thyroid releasing hormone (TRH) and Micardipine was carried out along with HBO therapy. His life was saved however he suffered from disturbance of consciousness.

HBO therapy performed 50 times and pharmacotherapy were undertaken on the patient in hope of recovery. A definite decline continued in the recovery, like changes observed in rCBF findings displayed through the continuous C15 O2 inhalation in PET images and in the changes in oxygen consumption detected by continuous 15 O2 inhalation. The symptoms were fixed and confirmation was made of them. While the patient had slight impairment with the possibility of color vision, he could see the objects but could not confirm them. There was positive verification on partial decline in functions that well substantiated the clinical findings.

Case II: Aged 65 years; male. The subject suffered CO poisoning from a briquette fire and was discovered in a comatose state. He completely recovered temporarily and was discharged from the hospital. However three weeks later he experienced a decline in his level of consciousness. It was a typical case of intermittent CO poisoning demonstrating symptoms of anischuria and grasp reflex. A slight decline in rCMRO2 of the frontal lobe was detected by positron CT using 15O2 whereas according to findings by C15O2, there was no change in rCBF. Similar to the previous case, pharmacotherapy employing TRH and Micardipine in combination with sixty times of HBO therapy was carried out. He recovered from the symptoms of anischuria during hospital visits as well as oneself, and aspasia, etc., as far as being able to cite his birth date. A rise in the frontal oxygen uptake rate, which had dropped prior to treatment, along with an improvement in rCMRO2 were observed by PET at that time. This was confirmed by PET as an amelioration in the clinical symptoms of cortical impairment. Looking at the changes in the cerebral functions depicted in the EEG topographic map, only a mixture of diffused low amplitude and slow waves was evidences prior to treatment. Recovery extended up to a normal EEG pattern. This case which was a CO poisoning intermittent type indicated dysfunction of the cerebral cortex.

Case III: Aged 68 years; female. This is a case afflicted with disturbance of consciousness following cardiac arrest revival. A hemorrhagic lesion was found in the left occipital region in the CT scans taken following cardiac arrest during a stellar nerve block in the outpatient anesthesiology department and revival resulting in motor paralysis and disturbance o consciousness. When positron CT images centering around the hemorrhagic region were examined, the defect could be detected in both C15O2 and 15O2 images where circulation and metabolism were found defective. The metabolic changes in 15O2 were unexpectedly mild and it was predicted that the tissues themselves retained some remaining functions. In such cases HBO therapy was performed 30 times. In the positron CT following treatment marked improvements were noted in the right CBF. It was believed attributable to improvement in the cerebral edema. Simultaneously, the metabolic region expanded on the left side. This was substantiated by improvements in the clinical symptoms of motor paralysis and disturbance of consciousness. In other words, even if there was a decline of perfusion in the cerebral tissue, it was found that rCBF and rCMRO2 could be improved in the early stages through the ameliorating effects of HBO therapy on cerebral edema. Furthermore, when a comparison was made throughout the course with EEG topographic maps, a tendency towards slowing was naturally observed in the findings. Corresponding to the hemorrhagic region, the presence of an area with low amplitude was witnessed, however its range did not correspond to the positron CT and was much greater than that viewed in positron CT.

Case IV: Aged 36 years; female. She inhaled H2S gas and had respiratory arrest. Following this, she had repeated convulsions. Her CT findings and clinical state suggested severe anoxic encephalopathy and continuous deep coma state. After repeating HBO therapy, with Nicarudipine, TRH and cytochrome C for two months, the patient gradually improved and became able to calculate. The changes in the region corresponded with the clinical symptoms observed with PET. It was confirmed that rCBF and rCMRO2 had improved and our treatment was useful.

DISCUSSION

The effects of HBO therapy on these three cases is summarized below.

Luxury perfusion syndrome of the basal ganglia is clearly indicated in the positron CT of severe acute cases of CO poisoning as in Case I. There was a region where perfusion was only high in the lesion indicating dysfunction (3). Recovery in such cases is difficult even with HBO therapy. In correspondence to transmigration to organic changes and becoming fixed, this progress is translated into clinical symptoms.

According to PET images, changes of perfusion were not found in mild cases of CO poisoning where no abnormalities remained in the basal ganglia region as in Case II. However in intermittent types which showed metabolic deterioration resulting from a decline in cortical rCMRO2 as depicted in 15O2 images, rises in rCMRO2 and wide range improvements in cortical impairment brought on by HBO therapy carried out 60 times were confirmed by PET. This was also verified in clinical symptoms and EEG topography. In this intermittent type of CO poisoning, alterations lay primarily in the white matter of the brain. With treatment involving mainly HBO therapy, pharmacotheraphy employing Ca++ antagonist Nicardipine and TRH demonstrated effectiveness.

Although there is a conspicuous decline in perfusion in new hemorrhagic lesions, as in Case III, in such cases with remains of cerebral metabolism, a recovery in cerebral circulation resulting from improvement in cerebral edema by HBO therapy was observed (4). This proves the efficiency of HBO therapy (5, 7). Patients showed coupling between rCBF and rCMRO2 as in Cases III and IV. Our studies suggest that HBO confers protections against ischemic brain damage. These findings have shown positron CT to be an extremely important diagnostic tool, surpassing X-Ray CT in cases that have been difficult to diagnose up to now by conventional methods.

CONCLUSION

(1) In the severe case of CO poisoning lying in comatose state with spasm complications, an enhancement of the basal ganglia was observed in X-Ray CT findings. Afterwards local abnormalities corresponding to the symptoms were confirmed by PET.

(2) Although abnormality in rCBF was mild according to PET in the intermittent type of CO poisoning, the regional cerebral metabolic rate that corresponded to the clinical symptoms was witnessed.

(3) Primarily HBO therapy along with TRH and Nicardipine was found effective in the treatment of CO poisoning.

(4) The prognosis for early detection was abnormal basal ganglia in the severe case of CO poisoning was poor, however the intermittent type was believed related to the white matter of the brain in which treatment performing HBO therapy 50 times proved effective.

(5) Distinct focal points of clinical symptoms that could not be clearly differentiated in X-Ray CT were revealed in PET and corresponded to abnormalities in EEG topographic maps.

(6) The decreased cerebral functions on the hemorrhagic side in the X-ray CT was observed in PET. Since the decrease was slight it was improved by HBO therapy.

REFERENCES

1. Jones, T., Chesler, D.A. and Ter Pogassian, M.M.: THe continuous inhalation of oxygen 15 for assessing regional extraction in the brain of man. Br. J. Radiol. 49: 339-343, 1976.
2. Frackowiack, R.S. Lengi, G.L., Jones, T. et al: Quantiatine measurement of regional cerebral blood flow and oxygen metabolism in man using 15 O and positron emission tomography. Theory, procedure and normal values. J. Comput. Assist. Tomogr. 4: 727-736, 1980.
3. Lassen, N.A.: The luxury perfusion syndrome and its possible relation to acute metabolic acidosis localized within the brain. Lancet II: 1113-1115, 1966.
4. Pierce, E.C., et al.: Cerebral edema, Hyperbaric Oxygen Therapy. Eds. Jefferson C., Davis, M.D., Thomas Hunt, M.D., Maryland. The Undersea Medical Society; p. 287, 1977.
5. Baron, J.C., Bousser, M.G., Comar, D., et al.: Noninvasive tomographic study of cerebral bloodflow and oxygen metabolism in vivo: Potentials, limitations and clinical applications in cerebral ischemic disorders. Eur. Neurol. 20: 273-284, 1981.
6. Baron, J.C., Rongemont, D., Bousser, M.G., et al.: Local CBF, oxygen extraction fraction (OEF) and CMRO2: Prognostic value in recent supratentorial infarction in humans. J. CEreb. Blood Flow Metabl. 3: Suppl. 1, s1-s2, 1983.
7. Baron, J.C., Bousser, M.G., Rey, A., et al.: Reversal of focal "Misery-Perfusion Syndrome" by extra intracranial arterial bypass in homodynamic cerebral ischemia. Stroke 12: 454-459, 1981.

Change of breathing pattern at 3 ATA

Tamaya, S., Makajima, I., Yamabayashi, H. and Ohta, Y.

Department of Emergency and Critical Care Medicine,
Tokai University, Department of Internal Medicine
Kanagawa, Japan.

3 ATA (Atmospheric Absolute) is commonly used pressure for hyperbaric oxygen therapy. At that pressure, density of gas increases three times, and partial pressure of nitrogen and oxygen also increase. Many studies have been done in the field of the change of ventilation at depth for the last two decades.

Lanphier found the marked CO_2 retention in divers under increased pressure breathing nitrogen-oxygen mixtures in 1963. And Schaefer found the same phenomena in divers during exposure to a helium-oxygen-nitrogen mixture at 7 ATA with an ambient CO_2 level of 1.1%. These findings raised the question of whether exposure to pressure alter the sensitivity of the respiratory centre to carbon dioxide resulting in a decreased ventilation or whether an increased work of respiration at depth is responsible for the alveolar hypoventilation.

Ventilatory response to carbon dioxide used to be a useful technique to evaluate a function of respiratory centre. But at increased pressure environment, minute ventilation will reduce not only due to a depressed function of the respiratory centre, but also due to increased resistive load to the airway.

With a newly developed technique of Pol by Milic-Emili and Whitelaw at Montreal group, it became possible to evaluate the central inspiratory activity (CIA) without influence by changes of pulmonary mechanics.

Linnarson revealed that the CIA increase despite the ventilatory response reduce at depth. The same findings were observed by authors during the saturation diving at 31 ATA Helium-oxygen-nitrogen environment in 1979. (Sea dragon IV).

Recently, pattern of breathing is studied using the equation of $Ve = Vt/Ti \times Ti/Tt$. Mean inspiratory flow Vt/Ti relate to CIA, and inspiratory duty cycle represent timing control.

At depth, CIA may increase, but its relation to mean inspiratory flow and timing control remain to be studied.

METHOD:

Five healthy adult male and one female took part as subjects. All have experienced a hyperbaric environment prior to this experiment. Breathing pattern was monitored for 30 minutes at 1 ATA and at 3 ATA.

Data of breathing pattern was collected for three minutes during the breathing rest. And the parameters of breathing pattern were collected while rebreathing was performed. These measurements were done at 1 ATA and at 3 ATA.

Two sets of measurements were done here. In the experiment I, inspiratory duration Ti, experiatory duration Te, and tidal volume Vt were measured for each breath, using hotwire pneumotachograph and inductive plethysmograph. Hotwire pneumotachograph was calibrated each time at the measurement with a cylinder pump calibrator. Electrical output from this pneumotachograph showed linear relationship with environmental pressure, so calibration factor became three times at 3 ATA. Inductive plethysmograph can evaluate the change of volume semiquantitatively within 10% of error. We compared the change of electrical output between 1 ATA and 3 ATA as % change.

In the experiment II, 10L of plastic bag was used for rebreathing. Five liters of 100% oxygen and 35% oxygen - 65% nitrogen were used at 1 ATA and 3 ATA respectively. Hey's plot, Ti, Te and Ti/Tt were evaluated while minutes ventilation was gradually increasing at rebreathing. Breathing patterns when minutes ventilation is between 11L and 13L were studied statistically. Paired t- test were used to compare the differences between at 1 ATA and at 3 ATA results.

In the experiment one, Ti was 1.56 ± 0.23 and 1.74 ± 0.31 sec. at 1 ATA and 3 ATA respectively. T was 2.12 ± 0.34 and 2.46 ± 0.48 sec, and R.R. 16.7 ± 2.4 and 14.9 ± 1.8, at 1 ATA and 3 ATA respectively. These changes were not statistically significant. Tidal volume measured with hotwire were 385 112 ml and 407 ± 125 ml at 1 ATA and 3 ATA respectively. This change was not significant. But the change of tidal volume obtained by inductive plethysmograph showed 28% of increasing at 3 ATA, compared to that at 1 ATA. Minutes ventilation was 6.42 ± 2.3 L/min at 1 ATA, 6.06 ± 1.8 L/min at 3 ATA (hotwire) and 7.30 ± 2.1 L/min at 3 ATA (inductive plethysmo).

In the experiment II, the relation between Vt and Ve which was calculated from Ti, Te and Vt of each breath was evaluated with so-called Hey's plot (Fig 1).

On this figure, white Ve is increasing, tidal volume was larger at 3 ATA than at 1 ATA at the same value of minutes ventilation. Both Ti and Te were prolonged at 3 ATA for the same minute ventilation. Breathing pattern in the term of Ti, Te, Vt/Ti, Vt/Te and VT when minute ventilation were between 11 and 13l/min are studied on the Table 1, where, Ti and Te flow changed much. Although respiratory rate decrease 17% and tidal volume increased 18% at 3 ATA, p value were 0.1.

DISCUSSION

It is always difficult to confirm steady state at 1 ATA and 3 ATA. Steady state at 3 ATA may be different from that at 1 ATA, because some accumulation of CO_2 at depth was reported. There is also inter-breath variability.

Minute ventilation calculated from each tidal volume may be variable in the range of 30 to 50%. Anticipation for the experiment also may change the breathing pattern. So we evaluated the changes of mean Ti, Te, Vt during three minutes of breathing. Although tendency of prolongation of Ti, and Te were observed, it is not significant statistically. Discrepancy in the measurement of tidal volume between hot wire pneumotachograph and with an inductive plethysmograph was observed. It is suggested that the discrepancy came from increased resistive load. Increased tidal volume measured with an inductive plethysmograh means increased pumping function of the thoracic cage despite the airflow measured with a hot wire at the mouth did not increase much. This finding suggests that there is increased workload on breathing even at the depth of 3 ATA.

The change of minute ventilation remains unanswered in this experiment.

In the experiment II, the change of breathing pattern was more enhanced by strong chemical control on respiratory centre by CO_2. With Read's rebreathing technique, slow and gradual chemical stimulation of CO_2 on the respiratory centre induced rather uniform breathing pattern which is increasing in the term of the minutes ventilation (Fig. 1). In this experiment, it was possible to pick up several breaths from which the minutes ventilation can be calculated between 11-12l/min. Inspiratory duration was prolonged at 3 ATA significantly ($p<0.01$). And expiratory duration was also prolonged ($p<0.05$). In the recent research, it is well observed that Ti is prolonged under inspiratory resistive load. Tidal volume may or may not increase under the same condition. And also, expiratory duration prolong under expiratory resistive load.

The breathing pattern at 3 ATA is the same breathing pattern under resistive load. Farhi and Maio reported that the maximum voluntary ventilation (MVV) at 4 ATA become one half of the original MVV at 1 ATA. Airway resistance at ATA become twice of that at 1 ATA. So, even at 3 ATA, resistive load to airway is considerable. It is difficult to know the relation between pressure and the change of breathing pattern at the higher pressure environment, because of possible change on the chemical regulation on the respiratory controller.

CONCLUSION

At increased air environment of 3 ATA, CIA may increase to compensate the increased resistive load, and to maintain the mean inspiratory flow unchanged.

Prolongation of inspiratory duration and unchanged mean inspiratory flow create deeper tidal volume at 3 ATA.

Increased end inspiratory lung volume and unchanged mean expiratory flow require prolonged expiratory duration.

At 3 ATA air environment where HBO is commonly operated, slow and deep ventilation is the pattern of breathing.

The mechanism how the CIA increase, and how the inspiratory duration is prolonged remains unanswered.

Table 1. Result II, Breathing pattern when VE is 12L/Min

TI (sec)	TE (sec)	VT/TI	VT/TE	RR	VT (ml)
Control	1.48	1.96	493	354	18.5	679
At 1 ATA	(.23)	(.34)	(120)	(112)	(2.3)	(232)
Parameters	1.63	2.33	494	345	15.4	803
At 3 ATA	(.36)	(.45)	(136)	(125)	(143)	(174)
Significance	p<.01	P<.05	NS	NS	P<.1	P<.1

(1 SD in parenthesis)

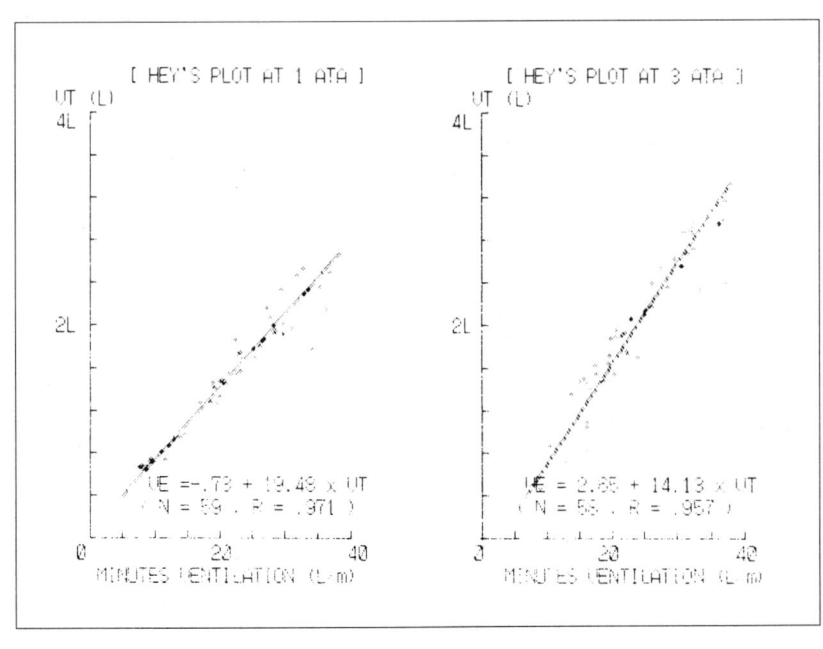

Figure 1.